Healing
Your
Child

Healing Your Child

An A–Z Guide to Using Natural Remedies

FRANCES DARRAGH and
LOUISE DARRAGH LAW

Marlowe & Company
New York

Published by
Marlowe & Company
A Division of the Avalon Publishing Group Incorporated
841 Broadway
New York, NY 10003
Healing Your Child: An A-Z Guide to Using Natural Remedies
Copyright © 1989, 2000 by Frances Darragh and Louise Darragh Law

The information in this book is intended to help readers make informed decisions about their health and the health of their loved ones. It is not intended to be a substitute for treatment by or the advice and care of a professional health care provider. While the author and publisher have endeavored to ensure that the information presented is accurate and up to date, they are not responsible for adverse effects or consequences sustained by any person using this book.

Library of Congress Cataloging-in-Publication Data
Darragh, Frances.
Healing your child : an A-Z guide to using natural remedies / by
Frances Darragh & Louise Darragh Law.
p cm.
ISBN 1-56924-614-9
1. Pediatrics—Popular works. 2. Children—Diseases—Homeopathic
treatment. 3. Herbs—Therapeutic use. 4. Medicine, Biochemic.
I. Law, Louise Darragh. II. Title.
RJ61 .D228 2000
618.92—dc21
                                                00-056853

9 8 7 6 5 4 3 2 1

Designed by Pauline Neuwirth, Neuwirth & Associates, Inc.

Printed in the United States of America
Distributed by Publishers Group West

Note

This book deals only with substances freely available in the natural world. We make no therapeutic claim for these substances. The body heals itself. We have presented existing information in a logical fashion for your individual convenience and easy reference. The reward we hope to gain is your recognition of the body's natural healing capacity. Being gifts from nature, herbs, homeopathic remedies, and cell salts can be powerful. When used with knowledge, their action allows the normal physiological functions to operate harmoniously and without interference. In some cases they are of value before expert help comes, while in others they can be of help during recuperation.

Contents

Foreword by Dr. Bruce Dewe   ix
Preface   xi

Introduction   1
How to Use Herbs   4
How to Use Homeopathic Remedies   9
How to Use Cell Salts   15
How to Combine Remedies   17
Resistance and Immunity   19

Common Ailments A–Z   25

A   Abscess 27/ AIDS 29/ Allergy 32/Anemia 35/
Anxiety 38/ Appendicitis 42/ Asthma 44

B   Babies and Nursing Mothers 49/
Bites and Stings 53/ Blisters 58/ Boils 58/
Breathing 60/ Bronchitis 62/ Bruises 65/Burns 66

C   Chicken Pox 70/ Choking 72/ Cold 74/
Cold Sores 75/ Conjunctivitis 77
Constipation 78/ Cough 80/ Cramps 83/Croup 84/

D   Diabetes—Juvenile 87/ Diaper Rash 89/
Diarrhea 90/ Digestive Problems 94/ Diphtheria 97

E   Ear 100/ Eczema 106/ Emergency Techniques 108/
Emergency Use of Homeopathy 114/ Eyes 116

F   Fever 122/ First Aid see Emergency, Fits 124/
Fractures 126

G Glands 129

H Headache 132/ Head Injury 134/
Heat Exhaustion /Heatstroke 135/ Hepatitis 137/
Hernia 140/ Hives 143

I Impetigo/School Sores 145/ Infection 147/ Influenza 148

J Jaundice 152

M Measles 157/ Meningitis 160/ Menstruation 162/
Mouth Ulcers 165/ Mumps 166

N Nose 169

P Pain 173/ Pneumonia 174/ Poisoning 177/
Poliomyelitis 181/ Psoriasis 183

R Rheumatic Fever 185/ Ringworm 187/ Rubella 189

S Scabies 191/ Scarlet Fever 193/ Shock 195/Sinusitis 196/
Sleep 198/ Spots and Rashes 201/ Sprains and Strains 204

T Teeth 207/ Tetanus 210/Throat (sore) 212/ Thrush 213/
Tonsillitis 215/ Travel Sickness 218

U Urinary Tract Infection 220

W Warts 223/ Whooping Cough 224/ Worms 227/
Wounds 228

Miscellaneous Ailments: 235
Bad Breath, Contact Dermatitis, Growing Pains,
Head Lice, Hyperactivity, Hyperventilation,
Penis Infection, Smelly Feet, Swollen Testicle,
Undescended Testicle

Remedy Pictures—Homeopathic   243
Remedy Pictures—Cell Salts   256

Bibliography   260
Suppliers of Natural Remedies   262
Index   265

Foreword

THOSE OF YOU fortunate enough to use this book are taking a giant step toward self-determination and freedom from the bondage of limited knowledge in child health care. When we become parents we want to do the best job we can. It is not until the baby is in our hands that we become aware just how abysmal our own personal training in child care is, especially in preventing minor health problems from developing into serious ones.

Today's young parents have great pressures placed on them socially to "do the right thing" for their baby. At the same time, social changes have resulted in grandparents being less available to assist with home remedies and other comforting advice when children are ill. Parents feel isolated and ignorant, yet don't want to run to the doctor with every little thing.

Frances and Louise Darragh are mothers who display a deep sensitivity to the health needs of the community. Their combined talents include naturopathy, homeopathy, Touch for Health, and One Brain Instruction. They are living and practicing the things that they are writing about. The result is an easy-to-use book full of practical professional advice. Problems requiring medical attention are readily identified so that referring to this book will not delay proper advice being sought in an emergency.

Frances and Louise have given parents easy signs and symptoms to help recognize conditions. They then draw on their professional knowledge to provide remedies for those conditions that are easy and safe to deal with in the home. Suggestions for seeking the appropriate health professional are also given.

Most of us feel we are just starting to understand child rearing when our youngest is finishing school. "I'd like to have known then what I know now" is a common comment. This book does much to remedy that and is the type of book I imagine that women of my mother's generation (born in the 1890s) could well have written, but didn't. We would have referred to it frequently when our girls were growing up.

The essence, then, of this book is its easily understood and practical help. It gives you the answers to a broad spectrum of conditions that form part of the "mysteries of child health." I learned things that have added to my capabilities as a parent. You, too, will learn things that, when put to use, will enhance the physical, emotional, and mental health of your children. The parenting experience will be less daunting and more rewarding.

—Bruce Dewe

(Dr. Bruce Dewe is a medical doctor who was for twenty years a family practitioner with a special interest in preventive medicine and health. For many years he has been the South Pacific trainer for the Touch for Health Foundation of the USA, urging people to take more responsibility for their own health care. He and his wife, Joan Dewe, M.A., have opened (1988) the Structural Neurology Centre in Auckland, New Zealand, dealing with chronic pain, fears, phobias, obsessions, allergies, dyslexia, and other conditions for which conventional medicine has less than adequate answers. Dr. and Ms. Dewe teach their work throughout the world.)

Preface

Dear Reader,

We HAVE WRITTEN this book because we have been in contact with many anxious parents who don't know what to do about their children's health problems. So many times, we have watched parents go off to their medical practitioner only to return with yet another round of antibiotics, no real understanding of what is happening with their child, and a lack of confidence that a solution will be found. We have also watched with grave concern the growing number of children on permanent medication, often requiring an increase in dosage and further medication as new symptoms appear.

We had been through this ourselves as parents and had turned to alternatives. Our partners, children, and pets have put up with some experimentation on behalf of our pursuit, but they benefited greatly in the end. In the early days, Andi went off to school with plantain leaves taped to her chin to battle school sores—experience has taught that there are ways of dealing with such things which require less fortitude from a six-year-old!

After eight ear infections in six months and almost permanent antibiotics, Kelly was of course on the list for the infamous "grommets" (tubes in the ears). Though herbs, homeopathics, Bach Flower Remedies, and dietary changes helped, any cold still produced an ear infection. We finally remembered that it had all started with mumps; homeopathic Nosode finished almost a year's neurosis and motivated us to write a manual for parents like ourselves, in search of alternative remedies.

There are, however, other stories—of Lee whose whooping cough seemed to respond rapidly to the natural approach, while her sister's condition steadily deteriorated despite our using the same methods. Her case of whooping cough demanded hospital care, and herbs could only be used to help her convalescence. Nature demands little, and does not always promise miracles.

We respect the need for many aspects of allopathic (orthodox) medicine. However, we also see a great need for caregivers to feel more confident and less useless in both understanding and taking measures to aid the path to health with nature's healers, which are safe if used as directed. The more you use them, the better the body will respond to their action and the more confident you will become.

It is not our intention to replace the services of the physician when such services are obviously required, but rather to complement them. With our alternative approach, parents and caregivers are guided through the progressive stages of illness and the journey back to good health. But if any illness lingers or is in any way serious (we give clear indications for this), it should always be checked and any actions taken monitored carefully by an experienced practitioner. Many medical practitioners are now willing to work with caregivers and can give you clear guidelines as to when the often more definitive action of drugs is necessary. If you are in doubt and feel concerned, the experts are there to be called upon. Be reassured—if used as instructed, natural remedies will not inhibit the action of allopathic drugs (although allopathic drugs may render natural remedies useless). Our hope is that the use of natural remedies will not only relieve the world's overburdened health services and save money for the family in the long run, but, more importantly, will give confidence and control back to the parents who are so often left coping with and caring for a sick child.

—Frances Darragh & Louise Darragh Law

Introduction

THIS BOOK OFFERS information on how to recognize and act upon children's injuries and ailments, by providing a comprehensive and practical manual. Information is given on the following:

- What symptoms may indicate
- The course an illness usually takes
- What you can do at home
- When to seek professional advice
- How to help the body through its crises in a way that complements any other forms of treatment which the child may be undergoing
- How to prevent a situation from deteriorating to the point where professional advice is essential.

HOW TO USE THIS BOOK

The main text takes the form of an alphabetical guide to children's illnesses. For the convenience of the lay reader and to make the vast symptom picture more accessible, we have compiled information under illness headings rather than specific symptoms. Where diagnosis may be difficult, information is listed under specific parts of the body. A separate section deals with resistance, epidemic diseases, and immunization (page 19).

1. For each ailment, we include:

    - The course the illness takes and its possible cause
    - Symptoms to expect
    - What immediate action to follow
    - How to make use of herbs, homeopathic remedies, and cell salts
    - When it is vital to call for professional help
    - What emergency steps to take before help arrives
    - Side effects, aftereffects, or complications
    - Follow-up approaches to help convalescence.

2. If you are not sure what illness your child actually has, refer to the index.
3. If you remain at all worried or confused, seek expert advice for diagnosis. Ailments of a doubtful nature or those that are not quickly alleviated belong under expert care, whether natural or orthodox.

USING NATURAL REMEDIES

Detailed instructions on the storage, dosage, usage, and combination of natural remedies are given in the following pages. Depending on which kind of remedy you favor, we recommend that you make up a health kit to have on hand in your home. Also look to any particular health problems in your family (such as asthma) and have remedies for these in your cabinet. To make your choice of remedy clearer with homeopathy and cell salts, we provide brief Remedy Pictures at the back of the book as a cross-reference.

FIRST AID

We recommend that this book be used in conjunction with a regular first aid book, such as that published by the American Red Cross. Also see Emergency Techniques (page 108), Emergency Use of Homeopathy (page 114), and Shock (page 195).

SEEK MEDICAL ADVICE FOR THE FOLLOWING:

- Stomach ache lasting more than four hours.
- Child is distant and confused, with dull eyes.
- Child looks anxious or in shock, pale or sweaty.
- Sunken eyes, skin lacking elasticity, dry mouth, and passing little urine (signs of dehydration).
- Neck is stiff and painful to bend or move.
- Panting, overbreathing, or deep rattling.
- Abdominal wall draws in upon breathing.
- Breathing difficulty is accompanied by blueness around the mouth.
- Blood and mucous appear in stools.
- Sharp object embedded in the eye.
- Convulsion or fit.
- Fracture.
- Soreness in kidney region (lower middle of back).
- Dark red or smoky urine.
- Coughing up blood.
- Coma—child can't be wakened.
- Sores that don't go away.
- Weight loss that continues.
- Blood or straw-colored discharge from the ear.

How to Use Herbs

HERBS CAN BE grown in your garden or be found in most health shops in a variety of forms: fresh, dried, tincture, oil, cough syrup, ointment, bath oil, lotion, capsule, or tablet. All forms are equally acceptable. Your child will quickly let you know which is preferred.

If you wish to produce any of these forms yourself, there are many herbal books describing how to do it.

INTERNAL USE

Herbs contain balanced supplies of nutritional supplements, with an affinity for particular body parts or processes; they work well when taken immediately before or after mealtimes. They can be used singly, but they also work well in combination with each other. Any amount can be combined at once. Hot drinks work best for colds, flu, and chest complaints. They also induce sweating. At other times, herbal drinks may be taken warm or cool. If desired, sweeten drinks with honey when lukewarm (over 45°C/113°F of heat destroys the beneficial properties of honey); if taste is disagreeable, make a syrup (see below).

Dosage: For best results, make up the required amount fresh each day and give 1 tsp. to ¼ cup three times daily. This can be increased to a dose every two hours in acute situations.

The total amount required each day will vary according to the constitution of the child. Use higher amounts for an older child, a stronger constitution, or a more severe disturbance; lower for a younger child, a more sensitive constitution, or more potent herbs (i.e., Hawthorn, Valerian, Lobelia, Jamaica Dogwood, Oats, Stone Root, Senega, Blood Root).

FRESH

For the light-textured parts of the plant (leaves and flowers) and crushed seeds, make as you would a pot of tea: 3 tsp. herbs (single or mixed) to 1 cup boiling water. Leave to brew for 10–30 minutes.

Alternatively, mix the same quantities of herbs and cold water, cover, bring to the boil and brew.

For heavy-textured parts of the plant such as bark, stems, or roots, make as you would coffee: 3 tsp. herbs (single or mixed) to 1 cup of water, simmer for 15–20 minutes, then strain.

Cold extracts can also be made by leaving the herbs in cold water (in a nonmetallic pot) for 8–12 hours.

DRIED

It is wise to replenish your supply of dried herbs every twelve months.

For the light-textured parts of the plant (leaves and flowers), make as you would a pot of tea: 1 tsp. of herbs (single or mixed) to 1 cup boiling water. Leave to brew 10–30 minutes.

For heavy-textured parts such as bark, stems, and roots, make as you would coffee: 1 tsp. herbs (single or mixed) to 1 cup of water, simmer 15–20 minutes, then strain.

TINCTURE

The suggested dosage is 6–20 drops (single or mixed) per cup of warm water or juice, depending on the constitution of the child and the severity of the illness. A rule-of-thumb for infant's dosage: one drop per year of age in a small amount of water or milk (up to a quarter of a cup).

POWDERS

Infants: a pinch to $1/4$ tsp. in a half-cup mixed with herb tea or warmed milk. Five to ten year-olds: $1/4$-$1/2$ tsp. in a half-cup mixed with herb tea or warmed milk.

A HERB HEALTH KIT

Barberry *Berberis Vulgaris*

Buchu *Barosma Betulina*

Burdock *Arctium Lappa*

Cayenne *Capsicum minimum*

Chamomile *Matricaria chamomilla*

Coltsfoot *Tussilago Farfara*

Dandelion Rt *Taraxicum officinalis*

Dong Quai *Shi di huang*

Echinacea *Echinacea augustifolia*

Elecampane *Inula belenium*

Eyebright *Euphrasia officinalis*

Gentian *Gentiana lutea*

Golden Seal *Hydrastis canadensis*

Horehound (white) *Marrubium*

Horehound-Marrubiun *Vulgaris*

Irish Moss *Chondrus Crispus*

Juniper *Berries*

Kelp

Licorice Rt *Glycyrrhiza giabra*

Lobelia *Lobelia inflata*

Marigold *calendula officinalis*

Marshmallow Rt *Althea officinalis*

Mullein *Verbascum thapsis*

Myrrh *Commiphorus molmol*

Rhubarb Rt *Rheum officinalis*

Rosemary *Rosmarinus officinalis*

Senna Pods *Cassia augustifolia*

Skullcap *Scutellaria lateriflora*

Tansy *Tanacetum vulgare*

Uva Ursi *Arctostaphylos ura ursi*

Valerian *Valia officinalis*

Yarrow *Achillea milefolium*

There are many herbs other than those we mention that are also of value. For practical purposes, we have limited our list.

HERBAL SYRUP

For coughs, colds, and the child who finds the flavor of herb teas disagreeable. Simmer herbs (single or mixed, using the amounts given above) until most of the water has evaporated. Strain and add honey when it is lukewarm.

CAPSULES AND TABLETS

These are readily available and directions appear on the packet. If not specified, use half-adult dosage for children, quarter-adult dosage for under two-year-olds.

EXTERNAL APPLICATIONS

POULTICE

The whole fresh leaf can be applied to the area and taped on. Alternatively, a poultice may be made as follows:

- Fresh leaves are crushed, bruised, or mashed with a little boiling water to soften; or half to 1 tsp. of dried leaves are mixed to a paste with bread, milk, wholemeal flour, and warm water to soften.
- Place the warm herbal mixture between two layers of gauze and apply it to sores, burns, bruises, sprains, or strains.
- Cover with a thick padding of towel, blanket, or hot water bottle to retain warmth for as long as possible.

COMPRESS

This is slightly less active than a poultice. Make a warm cupful of herbs using the amounts given under Internal Use above. Soak a piece of gauze or cloth in this and apply to sores, burns, bruises, sprains, or strains. Cover with thick dry toweling, blanket, or hot water bottle to retain warmth for as long as possible. The compress may be moistened with warm water from time to time.

INHALATION

Essential oils make the most effective inhalations, though strong brews may be made of fresh, dried, or tincture forms.

Add 1–2 drops of oil to a bowl of steaming water, drape a towel over the head to trap the steam, and breathe deeply into lungs.

BATH

Prepare several herbal cupfuls as directed under Internal Use and add to bathwater.

LOTION

Mix herb tincture (5 drops) or herbal oil (2 drops) with a quarter to half cup of Soya or Almond Oil (for dry skin, or as a chest rub); or of Aloe Vera (for irritated skin such as itchy bites or eczema).

CREAM

Add 2–3 tsp. of herbal tincture to 2.5 oz jar of aqueous cream. Especially good for surface irritations (calendula or urtica urens) or for bruises (arnica). There are now many ready-made herbal creams available.

How to Use Homeopathic Remedies

HOMEOPATHY IS A complex and comprehensive system of medicine. The advice we offer here is a simple approach for the lay person. If symptoms continue despite the use of the remedies we suggest, consult an experienced homeopath who can prescribe from the wide range of remedies through the complex procedure of detailed case taking.

Homeopathic remedies are easily obtained from health food stores and some pharmacists (see list, page 262). Some suppliers have a mailing system, so that you can order directly if you have difficulty obtaining remedies locally.

Homeopathic remedies work on the theory that like cures like, i.e., that a substance which has the ability to cause certain symptoms to appear when taken in large doses also has the ability to remove those same symptoms when taken in minute doses.

The remedies can be obtained in liquid form (alcohol-based and best avoided by those with liver problems like hepatitis or jaundice) or tablet form (lactose-based and best avoided by those on dairy-free diets or in whom you suspect lactose allergy). As you can see from their names, they are made from animal, vegetable, mineral, poisons, insects, spider's venom—in fact they can be made from anything. The process of making them involves serial dilution and vigorous shaking at each potency until minuscule potencies are reached. They therefore have none of the side effects of strong medicines if used in the potencies and quantities we recommend. Symptoms may worsen at first, as the body begins its healing work, but should improve gradually and consistently after this.

Homeopathic remedies are safe if large amounts are accidentally taken. If a child swallows a bottleful, it has no more effect than an individual tablet or a few drops.

Store remedies in a cool dark place away from strong odors. Because they are taken in such minute doses, their effects can be destroyed by excess heat or light, toothpaste, peppermint, strong gargles, camphor, and excess garlic, tea, or coffee. Do not directly touch either tablets or droppers.

HOW TO CHOOSE YOUR REMEDY

1. Take note of how your child has changed during the illness, comparing her to how she was when well.

   - How does she look? Anxious? Pale? Glazed eyes? Dry lips?
   - Has her mood changed? Is she irritable? Tearful? Averse to company?
   - Note other characteristics: Does she prefer heat or cold? Is she sweaty? feverish? thirsty? hungry? Does she sit up or lie down? Is she worse at a particular time of the day?

2. Next, using the contents list (and index for guidance if necessary), look up the illness and find the remedy that most closely matches your child's symptoms. If it is difficult to select one particular remedy, look up the Remedy Pictures (page 243). These provide more detailed information about each remedy, and should aid you in your final choice.

- It is not necessary to have all the symptoms listed under a remedy. Three definite and clear symptoms are often enough.
- If your chosen remedy causes no reaction after 3 doses, a different remedy may be needed. Retake the case, i.e., check your child's symptoms and check your choice of remedy. Do not change the remedy too often.
- Traditionally, combining homeopathic remedies with each other has not been recommended, although it is becoming more common to combine some remedies in low potencies such as 6x or 3c.

3. *Inimicals.* These are remedies that, in some cases, don't follow each other well and cause a negative reaction. They are Apis/Rhus Tox, Phosphorus/Causticum, Silica/Mercurius, Chamomilla/Nux Vomica, Ignatia/Coffea, Sepia/Lachesis, Calc Carb/Bryonia, Zinc/Nux Vomica.

Follow one with the other *only if absolutely indicated.*

A HOMEOPATHIC HEALTH KIT

Most homeopathic suppliers offer a first aid kit. A suggested starter kit might be the following:

Aconite	Ledum
Apis	Nux Vomica
Arnica	Pulsatilla
Belladonna	Rhus Tox
Chamomilla	Ruta Grav
Hypericum	Silica
Ignatia	

See also Remedy Pictures, page 243.

HOW THE REMEDIES ARE TAKEN

Homeopathic remedies are absorbed into the system via the mucous membranes in the mouth and therefore must be put into a clean mouth with none of the strong flavors mentioned above still lingering. For best results, take no food or drink (except water) for half an hour before and after taking the remedy.

TABLETS

Children can suck tablets until dissolved. Administer by tipping tablet into the lid and then directly into the child's mouth or on to a teaspoon and into the mouth so that there is no contact with the fingers.

For babies: crush tablet between two clean spoons and either place directly onto baby's tongue or mix with water on teaspoon. Do not place dropped or touched tablets back into the bottle.

LIQUID

Place 1–5 drops into a teaspoon of water or directly onto the tongue. If dropper touches mouth, wash it thoroughly with clean water before returning to the bottle.

HOW MUCH AND HOW OFTEN

30C POTENCY

In a sudden crisis: Suck one tablet or take 3–4 drops at each dose. Take a second dose 15 minutes after the first, then double the time between doses (i.e., 15 min/30 min/1 hr/2 hr/etc.), stopping the doses when the symptoms abate. From 1 to 3 doses is usually all that is required.

Stop the remedy if there is no improvement after the third dose. Retake the case, using the Remedy Pictures to clarify your choice and to see if there is another suitable remedy. Choose carefully—although the remedies in this potency are safe, changing the remedies too often can confuse the symptom picture, making later or more expert diagnosis difficult.

Acute illness:

Give 3–4 doses per day. Assess your choice of remedy after 3–4 doses by watching the body's signals; stop if better, continue if improving but lessen the frequency at this stage. Reassess if symptoms change or worsen.

For chronic illness:

Suck one tablet or take 3–4 drops in a little water, night and morning. Again, 1 to 3 doses are usually all that are required. In a chronic illness there may be no sign of improvement for up to ten days. Sometimes it can be seen much sooner than that. There may also be an initial worsening of physical symptoms—this is the body working—but look for noticeable improvement in mood and emotions. A continual and consistent improvement should then follow. If there is no improvement after ten days, choose a different remedy, using the Remedy Pictures as a guide.

After a month, if the improvement has stopped, another prescription may be given. Retake the case, noting the symptoms anew to decide whether to repeat the same remedy or to give a new one. Once again, don't give your child too many remedies as it may confuse the symptom picture for the future. Be aware that a single dose can continue acting for months if not interfered with by further dosing.

200C POTENCY

Give one dose in the morning and one dose at night in the one day. This is usually all that is required in sudden acute illness, some improvement should be evident within twenty-four hours. In chronic illness improvement may not be noticeable for up to ten days. There may be an initial worsening before gradual and consistent improvement.

If you are inexperienced in homeopathy, we advise that you use this potency only where we have indicated.

EXTERNAL APPLICATIONS

Lotions and ointments made from homeopathic remedies are available and can be applied to skin sores, bruises, wounds, or painful areas as directed.

Do not use Arnica directly on an open wound as it stings.

NOTE: Some people continually fail to respond well to chosen remedies. The information under Resistance and Immunity (page 19) may be useful here, but constitutional treatment is more effectively undertaken by an experienced homeopath or after detailed study of the miasmic remedies (which are not covered in this book).

You may find that one family member responds well to homeopathics while another responds better to herbs or cell salts.

How to Use Cell Salts

MINERAL SALTS ARE held together in the cellular tissues of the body in a delicate balance. They are vital to the proper growth and development of the body. An upset in the mineral balance heralds the beginning of illness.

Cell salts are prepared into minute quantities on a lactose base, and are easily assimilated by the body. When correctly chosen, they aid in restoring equilibrium. For those on a dairy-free diet, cell salts are available in an alcohol base.

We have included a brief Remedy Picture (page 256) for each cell salt to help your selection.

Cell salts work well in combination. However, they work best when alternated. Generally, no more than four are advisable either at any one time or (preferably) alternated at intervals throughout the day.

HOW CELL SALTS ARE TAKEN

Cell salts dissolve easily when sucked. For babies, crush the tablets between two clean teaspoons, drop water onto crushed tablets, and feed on a teaspoon. For children, the tablets dissolve very quickly on the tongue.

In sudden, acute situations:

1–2 tablets can be taken every 10–15 minutes. For a baby, crush a tablet in a small quarter cup of water and give a teaspoon dose at 10–15 minute intervals, increasing the time span between doses as severity of illness lessens. Discontinue when symptoms cease.

In chronic, long-standing situations:

1 tablet can be taken four times daily. If after seven days no improvement can be seen, it may be necessary to change or discontinue the cell salts. It is helpful to continue the cell salt(s) for several weeks after the illness has passed to ensure the original deficiency is overcome.

EXTERNAL APPLICATIONS

Cell salts may be crushed and mixed to a paste with a little water, then applied to affected skin areas.

RECOMMENDED CELL SALTS

There are twelve cell salts altogether:

Ferr Phos	Nat Mur	Calc Fluor
Nat Phos	Kali Mur	Silica
Kali Phos	Nat Sulph	
Calc Phos	Kali Sulph	
Mag Phos	Calc Sulph	

How to
Combine Remedies

HERBS AND HOMEOPATHIC REMEDIES

MINTS, GARLIC, CAMPHOR, coffee, strongly aromatic inhalations and flavorings can antidote homeopathic remedies so they are best avoided when taking them.

Herbs are best taken at mealtimes and homeopathic remedies a minimum of half an hour before or after taking food or drink (except water). If you wish to use them both in the same day, it is wise to choose those remedies that relate to the same symptoms. Follow these rules, and herbs and homeopathics will work harmoniously.

HERBS AND CELL SALTS

Choose cell salts and herbs that deal with the same symptoms. They can be taken together to repel invading toxins and strengthen the body during a crisis.

CELL SALTS AND HOMEOPATHICS

A cell salt may help balance the metabolic processes by enhancing the use of a particular mineral while the homeopathic remedy is working. In this situation you can combine them, taking the cell salt with meals and the homeopathic remedy in between. Corresponding cell salt and homeopathic remedies:

Calc Fluor	Silica, Kali Bich
Calc Phos	China, Ruta Grav, Calc
Carb	
Calc Sulph	Hepar Sulph, Silica
Ferr Phos	Aconite, Gelsemium
Kali Mur	Bryonia, Mercurius
Sulphur	
Kali Phos	Rhus Tox, Phosphorus
Pulsatilla, Ignatia	
Kali Sulph	Pulsatilla
Mag Phos	Belladonna, Colocynth
Nat Mur	Sepia, Sulphur
Phosphorus	
Nat Phos	Calc Carb

MEDICAL DRUGS

Herbs, homeopathics, and cell salts work harmoniously with the body's natural healing activities, and can in many cases be helpful while under medication, by relieving side effects of medical drugs without interfering with the main action of the drug. On the other hand, homeopathic remedies may lose their effectiveness in the presence of particular drugs, e.g., steroids, cortisone, some laxatives, nose drops, and liniments.

While the doses used in this book are within safe margins, if you are on allopathic medication for heart disease, hypertension or depressant there may be a risk of serious interaction. In these cases, we advise you to only use herbs in consultation with a Medical Herbalist.

Resistance and Immunity

ONSTANT EXPOSURE TO processed and chemically treated food, frequent use of prescription drugs, environmental pollution, and radiation all weaken the immune systems of our bodies. A weakened immune system contributes greatly to disease and poor recuperation. We can help our own and our children's immune systems by making appropriate changes to our lifestyles and by making good use of natural substances as described in this book.

DIET

1. Avoid foods that overload the system with waste products and rob the body of vital nutrients required to fight infection: chips, sweets, soft drinks, white flour and sugar products, fast foods, instant meals (frozen, canned, or packaged), excess meat, chicken, excess dairy products, and salty foods.

A note on dairy products and sugars:

Dairy products:

While dairy products unfortunately can create excess mucous and should be avoided if a child suffers from a severe runny nose, they are very nourishing for a growing child. Pasteurized milk is devitalized and more mucous-forming than raw milk. If you want to give your child milk, the most easily digestible form is as follows: take ¼ to ½ cup of raw milk, heat it to boiling point, add a pinch of spice such as cinnamon, cardamom, or ginger, cool and sweeten with honey.

Yogurt too has many qualities but can be quite heavy and hard to digest especially when taken with fruit (contrary to public opinion). The most digestible form of yogurt is diluted 1:1 with water, the same spices and sweetener added as for milk above.

Sugars:

Children need a certain amount of sugar for body building. However, if it is overrefined, it leaches the minerals out of the body. Honey is a very concentrated sugar so use small amounts only. Other excellent sweeteners are: maple syrup, rice or barley malt, and fruit concentrates.

2. Feed your children fresh food that has not been chemically treated, processed, or devitalized with preservatives, colorings, or flavorings: fresh or dried fruit and vegetables; sprouted seeds and grains; pure diluted fruit juices; homemade cookies, cakes, pastries, and breads made from whole-grain flours, honey, and cold-pressed oils; grains, beans, and unsalted nuts for protein, and herbs and seeds for flavoring; eggs from free-range hens; and meat and chicken from organic farms.

BUILDING RESISTANCE

HERBS

A general herbal tonic and cleanser helps strengthen the immune system and neutralize toxins. The following herbs cleanse the lymphatic system and also act:

As antiseptic: Golden Seal, Myrrh

To aid digestion during the cleansing process: Rosemary, Rhubarb Root

To cleanse lymphatic system: Calendula and all the above herbs

To detoxify the liver: Dandelion, Barberry

To help eliminate radiation and poisonous heavy metals: Irish Moss, Kelp

To help kidney action: Buchu, Uva Ursi

To purify the blood: Dandelion, Burdock, Echinacea

To relieve lung congestion: Mullein

To stimulate circulation: Capsicum

Choose your desired combination of herbs and make according to the instructions on page 4. Give daily for three weeks, rest for one week, repeat if necessary.

HOMEOPATHY

Homeopathic Nosode remedies can help the body rebuild resistance and help strengthen the immune system against further attacks. They may be used (1) if *during the actual illness* symptoms are especially troublesome or if complications set in; (2) for failure to return to full health after a specific disease; (3) if child has *never been well since being vaccinated* for the disease.

Take one dose (1 tablet or 2–3 drops of liquid) of the appropriate Nosode in the 200c potency. Give a second dose twenty-four hours later if there is no change.

Homeopathic Nosodes

Chicken Pox: Varicella
Colds: Bacillinum
Diphtheria: Diphtherinum
Hepatitis: Hepatitis A or Hepatitis B
Infections (constant septic wounds):
    Staphylococcin/Streptococcin
Influenza: Influenzinum or Bacillinum
Measles: Morbillinum
Meningitis: Meningococcin
Mumps: Parotidinum
Polio: Polio
Pneumonia: Pneumococcin
German Measles: Rubella
Scarlet Fever: Scarletinum
Tetanus: Tetanotoxin
Tonsillitis: Streptococcin
Whooping Cough: Pertussin

IMMUNIZATION

Those who wish to be thoroughly informed about immunization need to read detailed and well-researched information from those pro-immunization (available through government and medical sources) and those anti-immunization (available through health clinics and some health shops). "What Doctors Don't Tell You" gathers well-supported information on immunizations, their successes and failures. (WDDTY, 4 Wallace Road, London N1 2PG. Phone: [0208] 944–9555, E-mail: wddty@200.co.uk)

DO YOU PLAN TO VACCINATE YOUR CHILD?

If so, we suggest you choose a remedy from the list below to counteract any ill effects of the vaccination and to remove the residual toxins that may linger in the body and cause health problems now or later.

Homeopathics:

Give homeopathic Thuja 200c the night before and the morning of the vaccination, and another dose immediately after. If the child seems unwell two weeks later, refer to Remedy Pictures (page 243) and choose the remedy that most closely matches your child's constitutional type.

Cell Salts:

Alternatively, cell salts can be used. Kali Mur and Silica: one dose night and morning for seven days starting immediately after vaccination.

If, despite these precautions your child continues to suffer ill health after vaccination, the Nosode remedies may be given (see page 21). One dose of 30c or 200c potency is usually sufficient.

Occasionally a child will not respond to these remedies even when clearly selected. In these circumstances it will be necessary to consult an experienced homeopath, who is trained to take a detailed case history and deal with the complex total symptom picture.

If You Don't Plan to Vaccinate Your Child

If this is you, you need to be aware that you are taking responsibility for your child's health. We advise that you maintain regular contact with an experienced homeopath.

The homeopathic remedies given below may help resist invasion by foreign bacteria or viruses. In the first few days following contact with a disease, they can be taken in 2 doses of 30c for 1–2 days immediately after contact, then once weekly for 2 weeks, and once every 2 weeks while the disease remains in your community.

Chicken Pox: Rhus Tox
Diphtheria: Merc Cyanatus
German Measles: Pulsatilla or Pyrogenium
Hepatitis A: Kali Mur
Hepatitis B: Kali Mur
Influenza: Arsen Alb
Measles: Pulsatilla
Meningitis: Bacillinum
Mumps: Pilocarpine

Polio: Lathyrus or Gelsemium
Scarlet Fever: Belladonna
Tetanus: Hypericum or Ledum
Whooping Cough: Drosera

If your child still comes down with the disease in spite of these precautions, refer to the disease heading in this book.

CAUTION

It is important to understand that these homeopathic remedies may fail to act if the inherent constitution of the child is weak or impaired in some way. This may or may not be apparent, so as a safeguard homeopathy offers deep-acting remedies to strengthen a weak constitution. We recommend you seek expert homeopathic advice or have a thorough knowledge of the miasms before choosing to avoid vaccinations. (A "miasm" is an inherited disease stigma that can be responsible for the apparent variations in health among different children despite similar socioeconomic circumstances and dietary habits.)

Common
Ailments
A to Z

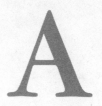

Abscess

An abscess is a collection of pus formed when an infection caused by some intruder is met by large numbers of white blood cells (to deal with the germs) and serum (to dilute and fight the toxins). This, together with increased blood supply to the area, causes redness, heat, swelling, pain, and tenderness.

WHAT TO DO—EXTERNAL APPLICATIONS

Do not squeeze. This is very painful and can spread the infection into the system.

HERBS

Make a poultice using a double layer of clean fine gauze, large enough to cover the abscess. Between the layers place your choice from the following: Comfrey ointment or fresh crushed Comfrey leaves, Slippery Elm powder (mixed to a paste with water), Golden Seal ointment, Teatree oil used directly or diluted with olive oil.

Place poultice over abscess. Cover with gauze dressing with a plaster. Wear overnight and repeat daily. When the infection has cleared, use Hypercal lotion for further healing.

CELL SALTS

A solution of the appropriate remedy (or remedies) from the list below can be used to bathe external parts by mixing three tablets with half a cup of reasonably hot water.

Usually, Vitamins A, B, and C will be lacking. This deficiency can be corrected by purifying the blood and detoxifying the glands. Echinacea and Golden Seal are especially helpful in this; Dandelion, Dock, Comfrey, or Poke Root may also be added.

HOMEOPATHIC

Anthracinum 30c: Black and blue abscess that looks decomposed.

Arsen Alb 30c: Burning pain, worse after midnight; better for heat applied to swelling.

Belladonna 30c: Sudden development, intense throbbing, bright red swelling.

Hepar Sulph 30c: Sharp, sticking pain, beginning with chills, tender to touch.

Mercurius 30c: Great redness with stinging pain. Follows Belladonna after pus has formed. Pyrogenium 30c: If abscess is swollen, discolored, and inflamed.

Staphylococcin 200c: For recurrent abscesses (for 200c potency, see page 13).

CELL SALTS

Calc Sulph: If discharge continues too long.

Ferr Phos: Redness, heat, pain, and throbbing.

Kali Mur: For swelling, alternate with Ferr Phos throughout the day.

Kali Phos: If discharge is putrid and foul smelling.

Silica: After swelling softens and pus begins to form.

AIDS/HIV

The following is a summary of information on AIDS as it relates to children. Because new information on AIDS is constantly coming to light, it is important to keep up-to-date if you are concerned for any member of your family.

DESCRIPTION

Acquired Immune Deficiency Syndrome is caused by a virus now called HIV. Having AIDS means that the immune system, which usually fights disease slowly, loses the ability to do so. The person becomes ill from some infection and, because of the HIV virus, general health continues to deteriorate until a life-threatening illness cannot be fought off.

The disease can incubate for a period of three months, so some people can have the virus in their system and not feel sick or test positive. Even after a positive test or the incubation period is over they often remain well and healthy for many years without moving to full-blown AIDS. They can still infect others, however.

The symptoms of HIV are not listed here as they are similar to a number of ordinary childhood illnesses such as colds, bronchitis, influenza, and diarrhea. We believe that to associate such typical childhood symptoms with AIDS would cause undue anxiety. What distinguishes AIDS is the duration of such symptoms, their persistence, severity, and their frequent coexistence with increasing general illness.

If you are very worried, there is a simple antibody test available that shows if someone has HIV. However, anyone seeking this test is advised to first read the information about it and to seek counseling to explain the meaning of the test results.

HOW IS AIDS SPREAD?

The HIV virus is difficult to catch. The virus is found in most body fluids (blood, semen, tears, breast milk) and in blood in urine, feces, and saliva. It is spread when the virus comes into direct contact with the recipient's bloodstream, i e., through cuts and abrasions.

Apart from the circumstances of sexual abuse, or contracting HIV at birth through infected parents, the possibility of a child catching HIV is still very low.

HOW AIDS IS NOT SPREAD

The HIV virus has been found in dried material, but only in extremely small quantities. To date no known cases of HIV have been transmitted

- By being near someone with AIDS/HIV;
- To nonsexually involved people living with someone diagnosed as having AIDS/HIV;
- To health workers through social contact alone or carrying out normal duties (however, there have been cases of health workers catching HIV, all of whom had open skin sores or needle-stick injuries and didn't take the precautions listed below);
- Through casual contact with older children or living with children infected with AIDS/HIV;
- Through casual contact like hugging, social kissing, or using the same cutlery, dishes, or washing facilities as someone with AIDS/HIV;
- Through contact with toilet seats, doorknobs, secondhand clothes, or anything else that has been touched by someone with AIDS/HIV. It is extremely unlikely (although theoretically possible) that AIDS/HIV would be caught by biting or being bitten by someone who has AIDS/HIV. Swimming pools treated according to the advised requirements are reported as prohibiting the spread of AIDS/HIV.

PRECAUTIONS AGAINST HIV

When assisting someone who is bleeding, if you have reason for concern:

1. Avoid contact with blood if you have open or unhealed cuts.

2. Use disposable gloves and afterward wash thoroughly with soap and water your hands, lower arms, and any other part in contact with or splashed by blood.
3. Place any cotton, gauze, etc., that has had contact with blood in a plastic bag and seal it for disposal.
4. Wipe down benches and other bloodied areas with cold or tepid water and then with household bleach freshly diluted 1:10 with water.
5. Wash with soap and water carpeted areas that have been splashed with blood.
6. Wash scissors or other instruments thoroughly in cold water to remove any blood, then sterilize by boiling in water for at least 10 minutes or by soaking for 30 minutes in household bleach diluted 1:10 with water.

Artificial Respiration:

Guards can be obtained from institutions and organizations. For accident victims *some* protection may be gained by using a hanky placed over the victim's mouth before beginning resuscitation.

Adolescents:

Young people need to know about HIV and the precautionary methods that help prevent the spread of all sexually transmitted diseases. If you have a teenager in your household, we recommend you obtain up-to-date, detailed information pamphlets from an AIDS clinic or your local Health Center.

Play centers, kindergartens, child-care centers, and schools should already have received material from the Department of Education discussing the above precautionary recommendations.

PREVENTION OF HIV

It is clear that some people are more susceptible than others to HIV, and many lovers of people with HIV or recipients of contaminated blood have not developed and may never develop the disease. A strong immune system is maintained by good health. Poor nutrition, physical and psychological stress, heavy use of prescription or illegal drugs, repeated and poorly treated infections, constant exposure to environmental pollutants and/or adulterated food all depress the immune system.

We can help our immune systems by being more aware of the above factors, making appropriate changes to our lifestyles, and by making good use of the natural substances mentioned under Resistance and Immunity (see page 19).

Note: Although it is not yet adequately documented, there is evidence suggesting that the condition of HIV sufferers has improved after they have dealt with the above stress factors.

In recent years, with the combination of medical and natural approaches, there has been good success in dealing with AIDS/HIV.

Allergy

A hypersensitivity to certain foods, drugs, chemical additives or vapors, inhalants (dust, pollen, grasses, etc.), insecticides, pillow and furniture stuffing, and animal hairs (to name a few) is an indication of allergy. For allergic reactions to bee stings, see Bites and Stings.

DESCRIPTION

The most common symptom of allergy in children is hyperactivity. Allergy can also show itself in any of the following: stress, schizophrenia, depression, fear, anxiety, claustrophobia, bizarre behavior, poor concentration and memory, bedwetting, vomiting, diarrhea, asthma, skin rashes, sinus, bronchitis, eczema, hives, local swelling or blisters, itching burning eyes, earache and recurrent ear infections, reactions to insect bites, trembling, headaches, abdominal pain, joint aches, strong cravings, flatulence, cystitis.

Note: Faulty metabolism and digestion usually exist before an allergy occurs.

Emotional disturbances may also be a factor.

Children usually crave or demand the food that they are allergic to. They will often throw tantrums when it is refused them. Once eaten, it will cause a temporary satisfaction as the withdrawal symptoms are relieved, but the metabolic system is placed under further strain.

TESTING FOR ALLERGIES

(Food, inhalants, or skin irritants)

Method 1: Pulse acceleration test
1. Have child abstain from the suspected allergen for five days.
2. Take resting pulse (i.e., sit quietly for 10 minutes first). Write it down.
3. Expose your child to the suspected allergen. If a food, preferably eat only that food.
4. A minute after exposure take pulse again. Write it down.
5. Take pulse again 10 minutes later. Write it down.
6. Repeat 20 minutes later (i.e., 30 minutes after exposure). If the pulse has increased by 16 beats per minute or more, this substance is a stressor to your child.

Method 2: See a Touch for Health instructor.
Any hypersensitivity is detected using a muscle testing process.

Method 3: Laboratory Tests
Ask your local medical doctor about these.

Method 4. Allergy Testing
A simple, noninvasive, painless and nondistressing test using a Vega machine. Appointments can usually be made at natural health clinics or shops.

WHAT TO DO

Allergies can be overcome without drugs. Carry out the allergy test Method 1 to determine what is an allergen for your child and choose any of these courses of action:

1. Exposure of the child (including the child in the womb) to many antibiotics or cortisones can produce overgrowth of the Candida Albicans organism. This can cause allergic reaction to yeast, marmite, yeast-based Vitamin Bs, wheat and sugars, especially refined carbohydrates such as cakes, cookies, and sweets. (See Thrush and deal with the Candida albicans infection as described there.) To replace the friendly bacteria in the small intestine, eat natural unsweetened yogurt and/or take Lactobacillus Acidophilus tablets (available at most health shops).

2. Eliminate the allergen from your child's diet or environment. When the system has been under stress from an allergen, the problem becomes exacerbated and your child may test allergic to a great number of substances. Don't despair. Eliminate the suspect foods from your child's diet for 2–4 weeks. You will find that after a time you can safely reintroduce most of the offending foods—you will be left with the original allergen. However, it is important not to become paranoid, as it is not always possible to avoid allergens, or indeed identify them in the first place. Instead, work on regulating the digestive function by adding spices like nutmeg, cardamom, fennel, and ginger to the daily diet.

3. Bach Flower Remedies are helpful for underlying emotional issues (available at most health shops).

4. Homeopathy has a corresponding remedy for most common allergens. Seek expert homeopathic advice or obtain these remedies directly from the homeopathic pharmacists listed on page 262.

5. See a Touch for Health instructor to rebalance the stress reaction to an allergen.

6. See an experienced natural health practitioner for difficult cases, as constitutional issues must be dealt with.

Anemia

A condition in which the circulating red blood cells are deficient in quantity or quality or both. It can be caused by excessive blood loss (rupture, hemorrhage, chronic diarrhea); deficiency in iron, folic acid, Vitamin B_{12}, or thyroxine; chronic infection or inflammation (by snake venom, parasites, streptococci, bacteria, chemical agents); hereditary disorders; kidney disorders; malignancy; or allergy.

DESCRIPTION

General tiredness, shortness of breath on exertion; giddiness; headache; pallor (especially of mucous membranes and palms of hands); palpitations; swollen ankles; indigestion; constipation; changeable mood patterns.

Additional signs that may be seen in iron-deficiency anemia: rapid pulse, thirst, sweating, sore tongue, irritability, heartburn, flatulence, abdominal pain, vomiting, slow healing of wounds.

Note: Skin color may be an unreliable test for anemia because of variations in thickness and pigmentation of skin.

WHAT TO DO

SEEK MEDICAL ADVICE. There are many types of anemia, so blood and feces tests are important to help establish the correct cause.

- Allergy can contribute to anemia by interfering with the absorption of vitamins and minerals—see Allergy. Sunshine, open air, and moderate exercise all help to improve the quality of the blood.
- Best foods are those rich in iron, B vitamins, manganese, and hydrochloric acid: brewer's yeast, green leafy vegetables, sunflower seeds, sesame seeds, almonds, bananas, plums, strawberries, grapes, peaches, raisins, apples, apricots, figs, honey, lentils, goat's milk, buckwheat, rice, beans, safflower oil.

- Best juices are green vegetable, carrot, and red beet, red grape, black currant, prune, and apricot. Take at least two glasses daily.

HERBS

For Hydrochloric Acid: Safflowers
For Iron: Yellow Dock, Golden Seal, Nettle, Raspberry, Rosehip, Basil
For Manganese: Black Walnut, Golden Seal, Watercress
For Vitamin B: Dandelion, Garlic, Kelp, Parsley, Chickweed, Hawthorn
To help build good blood: Red Clover, Echinacea, Myrrh, Licorice, Barberry, Dandelion
To help increase red blood cells: Gentian, Thyme
To help soothe intestinal lining in case of allergy: Comfrey, Slippery Elm

HOMEOPATHIC

Alumina 30c: For anemia at puberty with abnormal craving for indigestible substances, e.g., chalk, pencils.
Arsen Alb 30c: For pernicious anemia; exhaustion, edema, violent and irregular palpitations, craves acidic foods; extreme anxiety; irritable stomach, great thirst; looks weak and poorly.
Calc Carb 30c: For children disposed to obesity, catarrh, and diarrhea. Disgust for meat; craves sour, indigestible things; abdomen swollen; dizziness and palpitation on going upstairs; very worried about health.
China 30c: Anemia due to fluid loss, hemorrhage, diarrhea, too much menstrual flow; loss of vision, fainting, ringing in ears, pale, sallow complexion; sour belching, poor digestion, bloated abdomen; sensitive to drafts of air—better from fanning.
Ferr Met 30c: Bloated feeling followed by pale face and puffy extremities; mucous membranes are pale; easily exhausted,

may vomit food after meals; constant chill; maybe fever in the afternoon.

Kali Carb 30: Feels weak in heart region; backache; sweat; menstrual problems.

Nat Mur 30c: Good appetite but still thin and pale; throbbing headache, dyspnea (shortness of breath) worse from going upstairs; constipation, depression worse from being consoled; much fluttering and beating heart action; scanty menstruation.

Phosphorus 30c: Pernicious anemia; very tired, rapid energy loss, puffy eyes.

Pulsatilla 30c: Antidote for ill effects of too much iron. Chilly with gastric and menstrual disorders. Better in open air, dizzy on rising; no thirst; gentle, mild disposition.

Sepia 30c: Anemia at puberty due to irregular menstruation; severe headache, sinking at pit of stomach; constipation with ineffectual urging and passing only wind and mucous.

CELL SALTS

Alternate Calc Phos and Ferr Phos twice weekly each for six months if symptoms suit.

Calc Phos (helps to supply new blood cells): Face pale, greenish caused by poor nutrition; thin, delicate, pale infants; anemia after exhausting diseases. Waxy skin, headache, ringing ears, dizziness, cold extremities, heavy menstruation.

Ferr Phos: Follows Calc Phos as improvement sets in. Use for deficiency in hemoglobin. Pale face, flushes easily, pale lips; tendency to coughs and headaches. Ferr Phos is the normal constituent of tissues and is more easily assimilated than inorganic iron tonics.

Nat Mur: For young girls with dirty complexion; dry, scaly skin, constipation with very dry stools; palpitations; melancholy with bad dreams, backache, chills, fevers, and perspiration.

Silica: For long-standing signs of anemia in poorly nourished children.

Anxiety

This section includes behavioral disorders and learning difficulties. Anxiety is an exaggerated or inappropriate response to stress. It is characterized by feelings of anticipation, uneasiness, apprehension, or alarm often unrelated to anything or anyone in particular.

Note: In some situations anxiety can act as a positive device warning us against danger. Our concern here is with overwhelming or frequently recurring anxiety.

Anxiety can be caused by emotionally disturbing experiences, bad frights, encounters with hostile or disagreeable people; domestic strife; school phobias; lack of self-confidence; overwork; persistently poor communication with parents, family, schoolteachers or peers; feelings of being unloved and unwanted (e.g., after new brother or sister or stepparent). Can also be caused by psychological imbalances due to, e.g., lack of calcium; dietary imbalances; overdose of sugars or caffeine products.

DESCRIPTION

Physical symptoms may be palpitations, night sweats, tremors, diarrhea, frequent urination, headache, hyperventilation, stomachache, insomnia, nervousness, trembling, or fits.

Alternatively, the child may manifest undesirable behavioral patterns such as nail biting, temper tantrums, stealing, truancy, unmanageability, learning difficulties.

Note: While occasional incidents like these can be considered "normal" during a child's development, habitual, compulsive, or disabling behavior patterns need to be addressed.

WHAT TO DO

Rather than label these symptoms as psychoneuroses or personality disturbances, we look upon them as indications of a lack of balance or harmony between the body, mind, and emotions. While some children will respond favorably to the homeopathic approach, others may require Bach Flower Remedies to calm their emotions, or will benefit from nutritional improvements, especially in the form of cell salts, herbs, and the removal of junk foods from the diet. If you wish to follow these courses of action, seek further advice from a homeopath, natural health practitioner, or the books on Bach Flowers (available in most health shops).

There are also many techniques available to help us verbalize thoughts and feelings to become aware of how stress and anxiety affect us and our children. We can help by supporting and reassuring the child, and by making an effort to understand what the child is going through.

Sometimes it is necessary to balance the left and right hemispheres of the brain. To this end, there are many safe techniques available that teach how to balance mind, body, and emotions. These include One Brain, Touch for Health, counseling, NLP psychotherapy, and so on.

HERBS

The following combination taken daily for several months can help to calm the nerves: Valerian, Lavender, Passionflower, Vervain, Melissa, and/or Rosemary.

HOMEOPATHIC

Aconite 30c: For acute anxiety, extreme impatience, intolerance of pain, music, least noise; horrible fears; usually triggered by acute clear-cut cause (e.g., fright). Fear of crowds and open spaces.

Argent Nit 30c: Dreadful anticipation, impulsive, nervous; bites nails, tearful and apprehensive before ordeal of any kind; fear of heights, going to school, closed spaces, water, exams, stage fright.

Arnica 30c: Where there is a history of injury or fright; great fear with inconsolable anxiety and restlessness.

Arsen Alb 30c: Sensitive to disorder and confusion; can't sleep in a messy room; imagines burglars; dreams of darkness, fire, and danger. Changes place continually. Fears being alone.

Arum Triph 30c: Bites nails, picks at lips and nose, restless and irritable.

Baryta Carb 30c: Child is bashful, slow developer, acts stupid; doesn't want to play, prefers to sit idly in a corner.

Belladonna 30c: Imaginary fears, wants to run away. Delirious; violent impulses. Bed wetting.

Borax 30c: Dread of downward motion. Anxious and afraid of falling.

Calc Carb 30c: Night terrors; great anxiety and restlessness; visions of faces and people on closing eyes; school phobias; self-willed; insecure; always putting strange things into mouth, e.g., chalk, pencils.

Chamomilla 30c: Temper tantrums, whining, everything wrong, little things annoy; likes to be carried; can't bear pain; stubborn and obstinate.

Gelsemium 30c: Depressed, timid, anxious, tired, lazy, sluggish, worse after a bout of influenza; insecure, fear of failing, apprehension before an ordeal; tremulous and shaky.

Ignatia 30c: Stammering; feels effects of sudden shock or stress; depressed and irritable; bottles things up; dwells on problems in secret; bears grudges; sighs frequently; cannot bear pain or criticism.

Kali Phos 30c: Doesn't like meeting people; jumpy and nervous at the slightest thing; everything seems too much trouble.

Nux Vomica 30c: Frustrated, quarrelsome, critical, hypersensitive, aggressive.

Pulsatilla 30c: Emotionally upset and anxious, tearful and touchy, worse from bad news.

Tuberculinum 30c: Child afraid of animals, especially dogs; uses foul language, curses and swears; sensitive and dissatisfied; excited one minute, tearful the next.

Veratrum Album 30c: Tells lies, tears things, swears, inclined to run away; refuses to talk; sings, whistles, laughs, or acts insane.

CELL SALTS

Kali Phos (most commonly indicated remedy): depressed; irritable, bad tempered; sleepwalking, starts talking, wakes at slightest sound; timid, blushing, starts at sudden noise; exhausted from overwork; phobias, hallucinations, raving.

Nat Mur: Sad, apprehensive, negative thinker; hates being consoled, avoids company, easily annoyed; palpitations.

HERBS

Calamus Root: Helps improve intelligence, concentration, and willpower.

Gotu Kola: Helps improve mental power, purifies the blood, calms the emotions.

SLOW DEVELOPMENT

Occasionally the above disorders can be due to a lesion of the central nervous system caused by heredity, trauma, or environmental causes (e.g., meningitis, birth injury, malformation, deprivation of social stimuli such as deaf mutes).

These children will be immature and slow to develop, they may appear to lack intelligence and mental control, physical control, or have some form of spasticity or deformity. One Brain and Touch for Health techniques will be of the utmost benefit (see a Touch for Health or One Brain instructor), and it is wise to combine these techniques with the appropriate remedies listed below.

HOMEOPATHIC

Arnica 30c: Where a history of trauma has blocked the child's progress to maturity.

Baryta Carb 30c: For very slow psychological maturity.

Calc Carb 30c: Immature, withdrawn, exhausted, all life seems an effort.

Silica 30c: Stunted growth physically and mentally, leaving the child weak and vulnerable with profuse sweating and no physical energy.

Thyroidinum 30c: For stunted physical growth and very sluggish metabolism.

Tuberculinum 30c: Helps stimulate psychological maturity, especially where child is anxious and restless.

Appendicitis

Inflammation and suppuration of the appendix. Usually preceded by obstruction due to an enlarged lymph node and sometimes kinking of the appendix.

DESCRIPTION

Discomfort at the navel region that gets worse and worse. There may be nausea and vomiting. After a few hours this pain becomes sharp, shifts from the navel to the lower right side of the tummy, and is continuous and severe. Worse from coughing, sneezing, jarring, eating, and hot drinks. Constipation is common. There may be a rise in temperature (101–103°F) and an increase in pulse rate.

REBOUND TEST

Slowly press on the lower left abdomen. Release quickly. If there is a *sharp* pain when the hand is removed, appendicitis (or peritonitis) is very likely. If there is no rebound pain on left side, do the same test on right side. Again, sharp pain indicates appendicitis.

WHAT TO DO

1. OBTAIN IMMEDIATE MEDICAL ADVICE if appendicitis is suspected or for any persistent, severe abdominal pain.
2. Alternate hot and cold compresses onto painful area and continue with the one that gives most relief. (Hot flannel can be soaked in warmed Castor oil, applied to sore area and covered to retain warmth; or use a hot water bottle; for cold compress, wrap ice or something frozen in flannel and apply.)
3. *Do not give the child any food.*
4. *Do not give an enema.*
5. Over twenty-four hours give fresh, unsweetened fruit or vegetable juice.Best are lemon, carrot, apple, and beetroot. After acute symptoms subside, give a light diet for two days consisting only of fresh fruit, vegetables, soup, and Slippery Elm food. Gradually return to normal diet.

HERBS

As antiseptic: Golden Seal
To move bowels: Licorice and Rosemary
To calm and soothe: Elder and Slippery Elm
To purify blood: Echinacea

HOMEOPATHIC

Arsen Alb 30c: Chills, diarrhea, restlessness, and weakness accompany pain.
Belladonna 30c: Extremely sensitive to touch, cutting pain with fever, severe pain in lower right abdomen, pain worse from jar or motion, better from bending backwards. Useful in recurring cases.
Bryonia 30c: Throbbing, stitching pain, confined to a limited spot and worse from pressure, coughing and breathing, constipation and maybe a fever.
Lachesis 30c: Pain in lower right abdominal area, lies on back with knees drawn up, sensitive to touch all over abdomen,

worse from moving and feels weak.

Psorinum 200c: For repeated attacks (see page 13 for 200c potency).

Rhus Tox 30c: Hard swelling in right abdomen. Violent pains forcing child to bend double. Restless, better from hot applications. Cannot lie on left side.

CELL SALTS

Ferr Phos, Kati Mur, Mag Phos: Alternate these at 15–minute intervals on the first day.

Silica: Also give twice on the first two days.

Ferr Phos and Kali Mur together every two hours on second day. Kali Phos: Every hour if offensive stools accompany the pain.

Kali Sulph: If abdomen has drumlike sound on tapping, give every half-hour.

SEEK MEDICAL ADVICE

Seek medical advice if pain lasts longer than four hours. Although it may prove to be a case of chronic constipation or intestinal colic, peritonitis is a major complication of appendicitis, so expert advice should be sought. Peritonitis is rupture of the appendix causing generalized abdominal infection. A hard, boardlike tummy is the sign of advanced peritonitis and demands hospitalization.

Asthma

A disorder of the bronchial tubes (air tubes). Asthma is considered an allergic reaction, but infections, psychological and emotional factors are frequently involved as well. The bronchial muscles go into spasm and there is increased mucous production by the mucous glands. This narrowing of the air passages, congested with mucous, makes breathing difficult. Air is easier to draw in than out and the air trapped in the lungs makes oxygenation more difficult. If the disease starts in early childhood, there is a 20–30 percent chance of spontaneous recovery.

DESCRIPTION

Alarming difficulty in breathing (especially exhaling), creating a musical wheeze from deep in the lungs. There may be a cough. The skin has a bluish tinge. Attacks are most often at night, or early morning, and may last several hours or days.

WHAT TO DO—ACUTE ATTACK

We advise that you seek the help of an experienced natural health practitioner for this illness, as correctly used natural remedies can offer significant help to asthma sufferers, but we also advise that you use a medical practitioner to monitor progress.

- If your child is susceptible to asthma attacks, have something already prepared.
- These are immediate measures that you may find helpful: Place child in the position that makes breathing easiest—usually upright with back straight, leaning slightly forward. Your instinct may be to hold him tightly out of fear. Although it is important to reassure the child, give him breathing space, and remain calm yourself by taking Rescue Remedy or Aconite at 15-minute intervals.

HERBS

Tea:

Make a tea from your choice of the following herbs and have the child sip this frequently throughout the acute period.

To help relieve bronchial tension: Lobelia tincture (1 drop for each year of child's age—some children react strongly to this herb, so it is wise to begin with a low dose).

To help relieve spasms and calm the nerves: Lemon, Lavender, or Aniseed (can be obtained in oil form and added to tea in doses of 1 drop).

To help soothe the lungs: Comfrey, Slippery Elm, or Marshmallow.

To reduce the mucous buildup: Lungwort, Mullein, Elecampane, or Hops.

Inhalation:

Mix Lavender (3 drops), Eucalyptus (2 drops), and Thyme (1 drop) oils with hot water in a bowl and have child breathe this in deeply to help ease the congestion and tightness. (This process is more effective with towel over head and bowl to retain steam.)

Massage:

The above oils mixed with olive or Almond oil are soothing when rubbed onto the chest and spinal areas.

HOMEOPATHIC

Antim Tart 30c: For great rattling of mucous with pounding chest, worse lying down; child must sit up to breathe more easily.

Arsen Alb 30c: Worse 1–2 A.M., cold air, movement, or lying down. Burning feeling in chest, rapid heartbeat, great exhaustion accompanies the attack; better from bending forward, warmth, and hot drinks.

Ipecac 30c: May result from inhaling dust. Loose rattling cough, with gagging or vomiting but mucous does not come up. Great weight and anxiety in chest. Worse from motion.

Kali Bich 30c: Stringy, yellow mucous, worse 3–4 A.M., child feels better by bending forward and coughing up mucous.

Nat Sulph 30c: Asthma comes on with damp weather. Rattling in chest, worse 4 A.M., child must hold chest.

Nux Vomica 30c: Comes on after stomach upsets with belching and nausea. Worse in the morning and on a full stomach. Must loosen clothing.

Alternate Ferr Phos, Kali Phos, and Mag Phos at 10–minute intervals. If one appears to be more effective than the others, then you may give more of it.

To build resistance: Choose one or more of the following and have child take them twice daily for at least two weeks:

Calc Phos: Clear, tough expectoration.
Nat Sulph: Greenish expectoration.
Silica: Hay asthma, starts as itching and tingling in nose with discharge.

WHAT TO DO—LONG-TERM APPROACH

During absence of attack, treatment must be undertaken to strengthen the lungs, relieve mucous congestion, and build up the body's vital force so that it can withstand the next attack more readily.

- In some cases, misalignment of the spine can be a major contributing factor, as some dorsal nerves link directly with the lungs. Suspect this if the shoulder blades poke out abnormally, or if child has had a bad fall in the past. If necessary, see an osteopath or chiropractor about this.
- Always suspect allergies as potential causes of an asthmatic condition, either in the form of food or inhalants. See Allergy on how to deal with this. Consider temperature and climate in your region as these may aggravate the situation.
- If the child develops colds and infections, use treatment advised under these headings in this book to ward off possible attack.
- Check emotional stress. This can be a major contributing factor, so find someone who knows about Bach Flowers to help out. Books on Bach Flowers are available at most health shops.
- Take herbs rich in Vitamins A, C, and E such as: Coltsfoot, Comfrey, Burdock, Yellow Dock, Oats, Gentian, and Elecampane.

- Keep child's stress down to a minimum. These children are usually very sensitive to your stress levels, so keep yourself relaxed also. Relaxing herbs are Chamomile, Passionflower, Mistletoe, Lavender, or Lemon.
- If there is a history of infections, add Golden Seal, Southernwood, and Poke Root to the herbal combination.
- If the child has a tendency to constipation, add Senna or Rhubarb Root.

B

Babies
and Nursing Mothers

BABIES

HERBS

The breastfeeding mother can drink herbal tea and the benefits of the herb will be passed on to the baby through the milk. Alternatively, make a mild infusion of one quarter to one half a tsp. of dried herbs per cup of boiling water and give small amounts to baby on a teaspoon.

Using these guidelines, see individual headings for Constipation, Diarrhea, Sleep, Teething, and Diaper Rash.

Cradle Cap: Rub Wheatgerm oil, Apricot Kernel oil, or Castor oil on to scalp daily.

Infected Umbilical Cord: Apply a few drops of Myrrh or Propolis tincture after bathing and several times throughout the day.

Colic: Make mild infusion of Catnip, Chamomile, Dill, Fennel, or Ginger. Give in teaspoonful doses when rested.

HOMEOPATHIC

Homeopathic remedies are rapid in action and occur in minute amounts. They are very useful for babies—one drop in a teaspoon of water should suffice. See under individual headings for Constipation, Diarrhea, Sleep, Teething, Diaper Rash.

COLIC

Bryonia 30c: Irritable from least movement; can't stand to be soothed.

Chamomilla 30c: Often has one red cheek and the other pale. Cranky and impossible.

Colocynth 30c: Child doubles up with pain. Better from firm pressure on abdomen.

Mag Phos 30c: Colic better from warmth and gentle pressure on abdomen. Difficult birth or shock after an easy birth can sometimes cause the body great psychological stress, which shows in difficult breathing, color changes, limp limbs, sucking difficulty, etc.

Although births are attended by a doctor/midwife, the following remedies can be used:

Arnica 30c: For shock, bruising, limp limbs, difficult sucking. (Rescue Remedy can also be used for shock.)

Aconite 30c: Purple-colored face, shocked, frightened, or anxious.

Antim Tart 30c: Difficulty in breathing due to pressure and delay of difficult birth. Rattling in throat.

Carbo Veg 30c: For pale, cold, limp limbs.

Laurocerasus 30c: Breathless and blue, failing pulse. No rattle in throat.

FEEDING PROBLEMS

Aethusa 30c: Milk is vomited in large oily curds as soon as swallowed. Infant is exhausted afterward.

Calc Carb 30c: Hungry but dislikes the taste of the milk; these infants have large heads, large open fontanels, and a chalky coloring.

Calc Phos 30c: Infant wants to nurse constantly but vomits and develops diarrhea easily.

Mag Carb 30c: Colic. Intolerant of milk. Infant easily develops constipation.

Nat Carb 30c: Infant dislikes milk, which can cause thrush or diarrhea; abdomen becomes hard, bloated, and swollen, loud rumblings and pain.

Nux Vomica 30c: Blocked nose interferes with breast feeding. Delayed meconium. Child is restless and uneasy. Hiccups.

Tuberculinum 30c: Markedly worse from milk. Easy vomiting of milk. Very irritable.

INFANTILE JAUNDICE

Chelidonium or China 30c.

Wheatgerm oil (2–3 drops in the mouth daily) can also help. Skin problems can appear within the first few days.

SKIN

Arnica tincture: Apply externally to any bruised skin—avoid eyes and broken skin.

Arnica 30c: For bruising.

Calc Phos 30c: Bleeding from the navel.

Calc Fluor 30c: Birthmarks. This can also be taken as cell salt (6x). Thuja tincture can also be applied to affected skin area.

Medorrhinum 30c: For constipation with fiery, red rash around anus.

Phosphorus 30c: Moisture oozing from navel.

Sulphur 30c: Raw, chafed skin around anus.

SORE EYES

Aconite 30c: Red, inflamed, watering eyes.

Belladonna 30c: Red, swollen, and dry eyes. Worse from light.

Chamomilla 30c: Swollen and gummed-up eyelids. Often one red cheek.

Pulsatilla 30c: Swollen eyes with white or creamy, bland discharge.

Mercurius 30c: Red eyes and lids with yellowish discharge.

URINE RETENTION

Frequently occurs during first eighteen hours: Aconite 30c.

MOTHERS

HERBS

To increase milk supply: Aniseed, Blessed Thistle, Caraway, Fennel, Fenugreek, Rue, Vervain and/or Nettle. To decrease milk supply: Sage, Parsley.

To regulate milk supply and aid lactation in general: Black Cohosh, Ginger, Licorice, Marshmallow, Poke Weed, Yarrow.

To combat engorgement and breast infection, Vitamin C-rich herbs: Cayenne, Blessed Thistle, Poke Root, Echinacea. Ginger poultice applied externally. Make hot compresses from Comfrey leaves, Cabbage leaves, Mullein, or Lobelia.

For cracked nipples: Poke Root poultice. Rub with Wheatgerm oil.

HOMEOPATHIC

After-pains: Mag Phos or Cimicifuga Racemosa 30c
Exhaustion: China 30c or Cocculus 30c
Hemorrhage: Ipecac 200c
Pain of Episiotomy: Hypericum or Staphysagria 30c
Puerperal Sepsis: Pyrogenium 30c
Shock and Bruising: Arnica 200c immediately after birth

FEEDING PROBLEMS

Belladonna 30c: Breasts swollen, congested, hard and hot with red streaks. Very tender. Abscess.

Bryonia 30c: Painful breast engorgement, worse from movement, better from pressure. Mastitis.

Chamomilla 30c: Cracked nipples, cries out in pain, very irritable, and emotional. Suppressed milk due to a traumatic or upsetting event.

Lac Deflor 30c: Insufficient milk.

Lycopodium 30c: Sore, bleeding, and cracked nipples.

Nat Sulph 30c: Too much milk.

Petroleum 30c: Itchy, mealy covering of nipples.

Phytolacca 30c: Nipples sore with intense suffering that radiates all over body on suckling. Abscess.

Pulsatilla 30c: Too much or thin, watery milk. Pains extend to chest, neck, and down back. Suppression of milk due to shock or traumatic event. Insufficient milk. Also useful to reduce flow during weaning.

Sepia 30c: Deep, sore cracks across crown of nipple. Aversion to breast feeding.

Sulphur 30c: Nipple smarts, burns, and chaps badly; looks unclean.

Urtica Urens 30c: Insufficient milk. Swollen breast.

POST-PARTUM DEPRESSION

Ignatia 30c: Tearful and sighing a great deal.

Kati Carb 30c: Weak, irritable, tired, not usual self.

Nat Mur 30c: Wants to be alone; hides feelings but easily tearful; worse when consoled.

Bites and Stings

DOG BITES

If skin is not broken, wash thoroughly with Hypercal lotion (10 drops to half-glass water) several times over the next few days and watch for any worsening of condition. (See Tetanus, page 210.)

If skin is broken, clean it as above, and take internally:

Belladonna 30C once daily for seven days, then once weekly for six weeks. Follow-up remedy can be selected from the list below.

JELLYFISH (FOR DANGEROUS JELLYFISH STINGS, SEE BELOW)

Apis 30c: Give at 15–minute intervals 4–5 times.
Medusa 30c: If skin problems linger despite taking Apis.

BEES, WASPS

A bee stinger contains muscles that continue to pump poison into the skin, so the first priority is to remove the stinger quickly. Be sure to flick sideways with the fingernail. Make sure you do not press the bag as more poison will be pushed in. (A wasp has distinct yellow and black stripes and retains its stinger.)

Allergic reaction: Rapid, gross swelling starting at point of sting and spreading. Child often shows stress symptoms. Give Histamine 30c.

SEEK MEDICAL ADVICE if sting is on head or neck, or if sting is causing breathing difficulty. (Both orthodox and homeopathic practitioners offer a course of treatment to counteract allergic reactions.)

FLEAS AND MOSQUITOES

The occasional flea or mosquito bite can be alleviated with a dab of Aloe Vera gel or the herbs or homeopathics recommended below. However, numerous bites can cause great itching, irritation, and even infected skin.

- Homeopathic Staphysagria 6x once daily can act as a repellent during the mosquito season.
- When a house has been infested with fleas, Epsom salts sprinkled or Pennyroyal oil sprayed on the beds and floor will help prevent reinfestation.

POISONOUS CREATURES (SNAKES, FISH, SPIDERS, AND TICKS)

ALWAYS SEEK MEDICAL AID as soon as possible. If child is severely affected, apply Emergency Techniques (page 114).

Give Ledum 200c (2 doses over half an hour).

Pressure/Immobilization Method:

The purpose is to stop the venom from spreading through the circulation and into vital organs. DO NOT USE FOR RED BACKS, AUSTRALIAN PARALYSIS TICKS, BOX JELLYFISH, OR STONEFISH. (See below for these.)

Wrap a broad pressure bandage firmly round the affected area and keep part very still. This traps venom under bandage with very little escaping through the circulation. Make bandage as tight as for a sprained ankle and extend as high as possible toward the heart. Apply a splint to limb and bind firmly. Keep limb still.

Most regions have anti-venom available, so seek medical aid as soon as possible. (Anti-venom can be obtained in homeopathic form from some suppliers.) Try to identify creature. If this is impossible or unwise, don't clean the injury as the venom around the wound can often be identified for antidote purposes.

Red Back Spider:

Apply ice water in plastic bag to affected part (do not freeze skin) and seek medical aid at once.

Australian Paralysis Tick:

Remove tick as soon as possible. This will be easy in the first few hours, but when it embeds itself further, pour turpentine over the tick or lift out using a pair of sharp-pointed scissors. Do not squeeze tick; try to extract the whole tick in one piece, then use pressure/immobilization method.

Box Jellyfish:

Pour vinegar or acetic acid over adhering tentacles *before* trying to remove them. After five minutes, they will be inactivated and can be wiped off with a dry towel. Anti-venom is available. Use same procedure for other jellyfish.

Stonefish and Other Stinging Fish:

Seek medical aid for pain relief. Bathe in warm to hot (but not scalding) water to destabilize venom.

HOMEOPATHIC

If the poison has been absorbed into the bloodstream, the following remedies may be needed:

Carbolic Acid 30c: Very pale about mouth and nose with dusky face; foul breath, painlessness.

Conium 30c: Dizziness on lying down, turning over or least motion of head or eyes. Painful hardening of glands. Trembling, numbness, and sweat.

Crotalus Horridus 30c: Deathly sick, tremulous and weak with rapid serious development of symptoms; swelling with dark or bluish parts.

Lachesis 30c: Rapid onset of complaints with flashes of heat, excessive painfulness, especially of throat (must loosen collar) swallows often. Blueness of injured part with dark thin hemorrhage.

Oxalic Acid 30c: Numbness, weakness with trembling hands and feet. Livid coloring with great coldness.

WHAT TO DO

The following advice applies to skin affected by any of the above.

HERBS

Apply directly to bite or sting for relief:

- Crushed leaves of Plantain, Dock Mint, Marigold, Summer Savory, Basil
- Oils of Teatree, Sage, or Lavender
- Aloe Vera gel or Comfrey ointment

HOMEOPATHIC

Apis 30c: For bites and stings that burn and sting, for swelling about the throat and maybe the entire body; better from cold water, worse from heat, touch, or pressure.

Culex 30c: For lingering skin problems after mosquito bites.

Hepar Sulph 30c: Where skin becomes infected and sensitive to touch and cold.

Histamine 30c: For gross swellings or allergic reactions. Can be taken simultaneously with one of the other remedies.

Ledum 30c: For puncture wounds caused by bees, wasps, mosquitoes, or rats, where sensations are tingling, pricking, gnawing, itching. Worse from heat, movement, and scratching.

Pulex 30c: For lingering skin problems after flea bites.

Rhus Tox 200c: For itching and swelling that is better from warm applications. Use this remedy when there is no improvement from Urtica Urens or Ledum. Do not use before or after Apis.

Urtica Urens 30c: For pain, swelling and intolerable itching of bee stings. There may be puffiness, intense burning, redness and stinging worse on hands and face. This can be taken internally, but it also is safe to apply the tincture at 5–minute intervals on a compress when the face or eyelid are affected.

External applications: Tinctures of Arnica, Urtica Urens, Plantago, or Ledum can be applied together or separately to the bites or stings.

CELL SALTS

Nat Mur: First remedy for bites and stings, relieves pain, can be used internally or externally.

Kali Phos: If antiseptic is needed.

Kali Mur: Follows Nat Mur for subsequent swelling.

Blisters

DESCRIPTION

A raised fluid-filled bubble of skin caused by local serum buildup under the skin in response to burns (see Burns) or local irritation. Single blisters are not serious, but once opened are liable to infection.

WHAT TO DO

For any blister that starts to fester: see Infection (page 147).
For single blisters caused by local irritation:

- Sterilize a needle either by holding it over a clean flame for a minute or by soaking it in Hypercal solution (10 drops to half-glass water) for five minutes. Slanting the needle along the skin, slide it into the side of the blister to release the fluid serum. Soak up the fluid with cotton soaked in the same Hypercal solution.
- Choose *one* of the following procedures: (1) Cover with Calendula cream and bandage. (2) Dab with cotton soaked in Hypercal solution and cover with gauze firmly secured with tape or bandage. (3) Dab with Apricot oil mixed with a little Lavender oil.

BOILS

An infection that forms a sac of pus under the skin in a hair follicle, a pore in the skin, or a puncture wound.

DESCRIPTION

Starts as an itchy red swelling on the skin. The inflammation in a confined space becomes very painful and the swelling increases. A hard core of dead tissue then forms in the center of fluid pus. Can form in groups. Boils can cause swollen glands and fever.

WHAT TO DO—EXTERNAL APPROACH

Do not squeeze. This is very painful and can spread the infection into the system.

Make a poultice using a piece of double-layered gauze, large enough to cover the boil, and placing in it your choice of the following:

- Comfrey ointment or fresh crushed Comfrey leaves
- Slippery Elm powder mixed to a paste with water
- Hypercal lotion (10 drops to half-glass water)—dressing can be moistened with this mixture
- Golden Seal ointment

Place poultice over boil, cover with lint dressing or clean sheeting, and secure with tape or bandage. Wear overnight and repeat daily until boil is cleaned. When boil softens, core comes away with the dressing. Now clean with Hypercal for antiseptic and to help avoid scarring.

For bathing, make a solution of the appropriate cell-salt remedy: crush 3 tablets to half a cup of water.

WHAT TO DO—INTERNAL APPROACH

HERBS

Cleanse the system internally with Vitamin A- and C-rich herbs such as: Yellow Dock, Burdock, Poke Root, Queens Delight and/or Echinacea. Golden Seal is also useful for its antiseptic properties.

HOMEOPATHIC

Anthracinum 30c: Black and blue sores that decompose quickly and have black centers.

Arnica 30c: Crops of small boils all over the body.

Pyrogenium 30c: Swollen, inflamed, and discolored-looking boils. Better from heat.

Rhus Tox 30c: Red, swollen, and itchy; accompanied by swollen glands.

Silica 30c: Boils discharge their pus and do not heal readily.
Staphylococcin 200c: For recurring boils (for 200c potency, see page 13).

CELL SALTS

Ferr Phos: Redness, heat, pain and throbbing.
Kali Mur: For swelling, alternate this with Ferr Phos.
Silica: After swelling softens and pus begins to form. Also use after boil has broken.
Calc Sulph: If discharge continues too long.
Kali Phos: If discharge looks and smells foul.

LONG-TERM APPROACH

Boils indicate an underlying toxic condition of the blood. Recurring boils may be due to fatigue, excess consumption of refined foods (white flour, sugar products, etc.), poor elimination, faulty hygiene, or stress. Take steps to deal with these factors. Cleanse the system with the herbs listed above made into a tea and taken daily for one month. Also Staphylococcin 200c may be taken for recurring boils (see page 13 for 200c potency).

SEEK MEDICAL ADVICE if inflammation continues and spreads.

Breathing

RESCUE BREATHING

Breathing is essential to life. If a child is not breathing, this function must be restored immediately—before any other injury is attended to.

1. Place child on his back on a hard surface. Remove obvious obstructions—plastic bag, tongue, etc. Turn head to one side to remove vomit, etc.
2. Clear airways. Support nape of neck and press top of the head so that the head is tilted backwards with the chin up.
3. Loosen tight clothing at neck and waist.
4. Lift jaw and give 3–4 quick breaths into child's mouth while gently pinching nose shut.

ARTIFICIAL RESPIRATION

If breathing does not return automatically after above procedure, begin artificial respiration.

1. Open your mouth wide and take a deep breath.
2. For infants under 2 years old, seal your lips round child's mouth and nose, keeping his head tilted back. (If in doubt regarding hygiene, it is wise to place a tissue between your mouth and the child's.) Older children should be treated mouth-to-mouth gently, but like adults.
3. Blow gently into child's lungs until chest rises.
4. Remove your mouth and watch chest fall.
5. Repeat until help arrives or until automatic breathing returns. If head is well tilted back and chest does not rise, there is an obstruction. Turn child on his side and thump the back. Check for and remove any matter at the back of the throat.

Difficulties in breathing may be caused by the following (where appropriate, see under illness heading for what to do):

Asphyxia: Lack of oxygen, irregular breathing, blue/purplish skin color (if there is also no pulse, see page 110).
Asthma: Difficulty, especially in breathing out; usually causes a wheeze from deep in the lungs.
Bronchitis: Fever, sore throat, hacking cough, and rattling breathing.
Chest Cramp.

Cold: Breathing difficulty caused by blocked nose. (When infection spreads to chest, this is bronchitis.)

Croup: Difficulty in getting air in and out; husky voice; dry, barking cough.

Dehydration: Rapid, deep breathing; skin does not rebound when pinched.

Diphtheria: Generally unwell; sore throat, mild fever, hacking cough; foul breath—throat membrane has gray glistening appearance and bleeds when wiped.

Hyperventilation: Abnormally rapid breathing. Dizziness and lowering of blood pressure (see Miscellaneous Ailments, page 235).

Obstruction: Caused by objects. See Choking, page 72. Start rescue breathing procedure as below.

Poisons: Inhaled, e.g., ammonia. See Poisons.

Pneumonia: Rapid, shallow breathing; high temperature; pain in chest.

Shock: Shallow, rapid breathing associated with pale, cold, clammy skin. See Shock.

Bronchitis

Acute inflammation of the bronchial tubes (air passages of the lungs) that begins as an upper respiratory tract infection.

DESCRIPTION

Fever, hacking cough, sore throat; may be difficult breathing; pain in lungs or back, rattling sound in chest.

WHAT TO DO

Best foods are fresh fruits and vegetables. Avoid dairy products, sweets, and wheat products as these can create excess mucous.

HERBS

Make a tea, combining your choice of the following:

For fever: Lemon Balm, Elder Flower, or Boneset.
To loosen and help remove phlegm: Comfrey, Elecampane, Mullein, or Hyssop.
To purify the blood: Red Clover, Thyme, or Poke Root.
To soothe the inflamed surfaces: Licorice, Marshmallow, or Slippery Elm.

Inhalation:

Two drops of Thyme, Lemon, and/or Peppermint oils can be added to steaming water. Cover head and bowl with towel and breathe in the steam to clear the air passages and loosen mucous.

Chest Rub:

Two drops of Thyme, Teatree, and/or Clove oil can be mixed with a half-cup of Olive or Soya oil and rubbed on chest several times daily.

Bath:

The same oils can be added to bathwater (footbath is beneficial).

HOMEOPATHIC

Aconite 30c: Hoarse, dry cough; frequent sneezing; loud breathing; short of breath with anxiety and restless sleep. Use at first stage of illness and fever.
Antim Tart 30c: Rattling chest but very little mucous is raised. Child may be wheezing, drowsy, and feels worse from drinking milk or lying down. Must sit up to breathe.
Bryonia 30c: Dry cough, needs to breathe deeply, worse from motion, better while resting; stitching pain in sides of chest. Must sit up to cough.
Hepar Sulph 30c: Loose, rattling moist cough, hoarse voice, yellow expectoration. Worse from cold, touch, or least uncovering.

Kali Bich 30c: Tough mucous, thick and stringy, difficult to raise. Worse in morning, worse eating. Often accompanied by swollen glands.

Phosphorus 30c: Tickling cough; hot, tight chest; trembling during cough; pain as if something were torn loose in chest; worse from talking or laughing, cold air, touch, exertion. Better from dark and sleep. Use Phosphorus also for head colds that tend to go to the chest, and for lingering cases.

Pulsatilla 30c: Loose, thick, yellow-green mucous may be coughed up. Cough tends to be dry in the evening and loose in the morning. Pressure and soreness of chest.

CELL SALTS

Ferr Phos: For first stage with heat, fever, cough with no mucous. Give frequently for first 24 hours, then when cough loosens alternate with Kali Mur.

Kali Mur: Thick, white and loose mucous may be coughed up.

Kali Sulph: Copious discharge of yellow, green mucous. Continue to alternate this with Ferr Phos while there is a fever.

Silica: Thick, yellow, heavy mucous is coughed up. Worse from cold drinks, better from warm drinks.

CHRONIC BRONCHITIS

Chronic Bronchitis is indicated where there are repeated attacks.

- Use the above herbs regularly for 2 or 3 weeks. These herbs are rich in Vitamin A and are much needed to help strengthen the lungs.
- Also use the appropriate cell salt twice daily for several weeks but include Ferr Phos to oxygenate the lungs.
- Tuberculinum 200c: This is useful when response to homeopathic treatment is poor. Thick, easy expectoration. Craves cold air. Short of breath. (For 200c potency, see page 13).

Note: Make sure the child is not exposed to cigarette smoke (yours or anyone else's). This can be as bad for her as if she were smoking herself.

Bruises

Mechanical damage to the blood vessels or muscles beneath the skin without breaking skin surface. When damage is done to deeper layers without breaking the skin, this is considered a contused wound (see Wounds).

WHAT TO DO

HERBS

Make poultice using clean double-layered gauze large enough to cover bruised area. Place in it any of the following: Comfrey ointment or fresh crushed Comfrey leaves; Arnica ointment; Slippery Elm powder mixed to a paste with a little water. Place poultice against bruised area, place second, larger piece of gauze or sheeting on top, and secure with tape or bandage.

HOMEOPATHIC

Arnica 30c: Initially for all bruising.
Hypericum 30c: Nerve or spinal bruises. Very painful injuries. Crush injuries.
Rhus Tox 30c: Damage to muscle, ligaments, or tendons.
Ruta Grav 30c: Bone and eye injuries.

External application: Moistened, crushed tablets can also be applied with lint dressing and bandage.

Burns

Damage to body tissues caused by exposure to excess heat. This may be due to fire, flame, electric current, sun rays, steam, abrasions, caustic substances, dry ice, boiling liquid, tar or oil, friction.

Dangers from burns are circulatory collapse from pain; shock; serum loss (fluid seeping out from the burned surface can deplete the body of vital proteins, salt, and water); and infection.

DESCRIPTION

MAJOR BURNS

- More than 10 percent of the body surface is burned. The larger the area burned the greater the effect on the circulation and the more seriously ill the child will be.
- Destruction of full thickness of the skin. Fat and muscles are burned. Burns have a yellow-white appearance. The area is often not painful as nerve endings are destroyed.
- All burns around joints should also be treated as major.

MINOR BURNS

- Damage to outer skin layers only. Red and painful. May be blisters.

WHAT TO DO

1. Run cold water gently over burned area for at least ten minutes or until burning sensation ceases. Continue further procedures as necessary see below.
2. Give Arnica 200c or Rescue Remedy (4 drops on tongue).
3. For major burns: CALL AMBULANCE OR DOCTOR IMMEDIATELY.
4. Lay child down, cover larger burns with clean sheeting (diaper or pillowcase will do).

5. Keep child warm but do not overheat.
6. Give frequent small drinks of water (unless unconscious). Rescue Remedy or Arnica (4 drops to half-glass of water) can be added to this or can be placed directly onto tongue or lips.
7. Reassure frequently.

Scalding Clothes:

If clothes hold scalding or corrosive liquid, do not remove any clothing that is already stuck to the skin and pulling skin away, nor if skin is black and sticky. Instead, keep skin and clothes soaking and call doctor and ambulance immediately.

Acid Burns:

Bathe burn in mixture of bicarbonate of soda (baking soda) and water (2 tsp. to 4¼ cups or approximately 1 packet to a bath for larger burns).

Burns from Sodium Hydroxide, Ammonia, or Calcium Oxide:

Immediately put in water, then as soon as possible bathe burn in equal parts vinegar (or lemon juice) and water.

If Clothes Catch Fire:

Smother flames by wrapping rug, blanket, or coat around child. Roll on ground to help put out flames: douse smoldering clothes and child with water.

Burns from Electric Current:

After electric shock, child will either be thrown clear or go into muscle spasm and may remain attached to source. *Do not endanger yourself.* Cut off current at main circuit breaker or push child off using *wooden* handled broom. Check breathing. Burns will show only at entry and exit points of current and may appear minor. Electric current causes damage along the whole length of the path traveled, internal and external. *Always seek medical help.*

Sunburn:

If sun exposure has caused burning, use procedures as indicated below to help prevent potential skin problems (see also page 116).

IMPORTANT POINTS

- Do not endanger yourself
- Do not remove anything stuck to injury (including clothing)
- Do not break blisters
- Do not remove loose skin
- Do not apply lotions, ointments, fatty substances, or use adhesive dressings on major burns
- Always apply cold water as above—to this can be added 4 drops per cupful of Hypercal lotion as a lotion to wash the area clean with.

INTERNAL PROCEDURE FOR ALL BURNS

HOMEOPATHIC

Arnica 200c: For shock, three times in one day. For major burns follow with Arnica 30c 4–5 times daily for a few days if necessary.

Cantharis 30c: For raw, smarting pain of burns and scalds. To calm and help relieve pain. Give every 10–15 minutes for the first hour, then as needed.

Causticum 30c: For painful burns that do not heal, that fester, or that break out after having healed.

CELL SALTS

Ferr Phos: First remedy to give for burns.

Kali Mur: For deep burns and blisters, alternate this remedy with Ferr Phos at 15–minute intervals and gradually increase the time span between remedies.

Calc Sulph: For burns that appear infected or if healing is slow.

EXTERNAL APPLICATIONS

Any of the following will soothe the burned surface of minor burns and complete the healing of major burns after critical period has passed: Calendula cream, Urtica Urens ointment or tincture, Aloe

Vera gel, Vitamin E oil squeezed from capsule, liquid Honey, Comfrey or Chickweed ointment or leaves.

Ointments can be applied directly to burn and covered with cloth or bandage. Tinctures (5 drops to half-cup of water) can be used to moisten cloth or bandage to cover the burned area lightly.

SEEK MEDICAL ADVICE

- For all deep burns
- For all burns covering more than 10 percent of body surface
- For burns to mouth or throat, because swelling of the throat tissues can interfere with breathing
- For large or numerous burns
- For all burns around joints
- For all burns from electrical currents
- If pus forms on the burned surface

PREVENTION

Most burns can be prevented. Take special care.

- Do not let babies or young children go near a fire.
- Keep matches, lamps, and heaters out of reach.
- Turn handles of pots on stove so children can't reach them.
- Use short cords on electric kettles and have these in a holder so they can't be tipped over.
- Use nonflammable clothing.
- Always check water temperature before putting child in bath.
- Play safe with the sun. Avoid excessive sun exposure, especially for fair-skinned children and at the beginning of the season. Use sunblock.

C

Chicken Pox

An infectious disease transferred by droplets from mouth or nose. Shingles (Herpes Zoster) in an older person is often a source of contact. Usually a mild disease with characteristic skin eruptions; occasionally a child is very ill with it.

DESCRIPTION

Begins as itchy, red spots like flea bites, usually on the trunk. The spots enlarge, fill with fluid, and turn to blisters. These eventually burst and develop into itchy scabs. There is some discomfort and fever, loss of appetite and irritability. Common age for disease is under ten years, common season is autumn and winter.

Incubation period: about 15–20 days.
Isolation period: one week from the first sign of rash.
Recovery time: about two weeks.

WHAT TO DO

Keep the skin clean with frequent baths or showers, using Pine oil soap or 2 tablespoons of baking soda in the bath. Mix 3 drops of Lavender oil with 2 teaspoons of Olive or Soya oil and rub on affected skin.

HERBS

Good herbs for itch:

Burdock and Sarsaparilla. Soak a cloth in an infusion made from these herbs, or add it to the bathwater.

To calm itch:

Yarrow, Chamomile, and/or Lavender can be added to above herbs. They can also be drunk together as a tea.

HOMEOPATHIC

After suspected contact: Rhus Tox 30c may help the child's resistance to the disease when given night and morning for three days (starting within two days of contact), then one dose per week for two weeks.

Antim Tart 30c: For early stages, spots slow in appearing, with bronchitis, sweats easily, is drowsy and peevish but wants company.

Pulsatilla 30c: Weepy child who is not thirsty despite fever.

Rhus Tox 30c: Itching is extreme, mental and physical restlessness.

Varicella 200c (Nosode, see page 21): To help clear a severe case or for lingering aftereffects of the disease. *Do not give while disease is incubating.*

CELL SALTS

Ferr Phos: When fever, irritability, and discomfort are present.

Kali Mur: Alternate with Ferr Phos when fever stage is passing. One dose of each every two hours for the first few days.

Calc Sulph: Where eruptions have yellow infected-looking discharge.

To strengthen the immune system and help restore to full health after the disease or vaccination, see Resistance and Immunity, page 19.

Choking

Child's airways are partially or totally blocked by an obstruction, making breathing difficult or impossible. May occur when something goes down windpipe rather than food passage; when food is inadequately chewed and quickly swallowed; or when child has put something in his/her mouth and accidentally swallowed it.

DESCRIPTION

Difficulty in breathing; child will be unable to speak and may be gripping the throat; lips and mouth become blue; veins of face and neck become prominent.

WHAT TO DO

1. Remove any obvious obstruction to airways if possible.
2. *Baby:* Hold upside-down by the legs and give 3–4 smart knocks between shoulder blades using the heel of your hand. Take care not to hit too hard. If still choking, keeping head lower than body, place two fingers on center of chest between the nipples and press down ¼–½ inch about 4 times. Repeat if necessary. If this does not dislodge the obstruction, see #4 below for older child. Be careful not to use too much pressure.
3. *Toddler:* Put child head-down across your arm or knee and, using the heel of your hand, give 4 knocks to the back between the shoulder blades. If still choking, turn child over, keeping head lower than body, place the heel of one hand on center of the chest just below the nipples and press down

$^1/_2$–$^3/_4$ inch 4 times. Repeat if necessary. If this does not dislodge the obstruction, see #4 below. Be careful not to use too much pressure.

4. *Older Child:* Hug child from behind, using a clenched fist, applying sharp pressure just below front ribs to force the air upward and the object out.

HERBS

Scratchy throat: Gargle with strong Sage tea.

HOMEOPATHIC

Antim Tart 30c: Drowsy and sweaty, whole body trembles; great faintness, palpitation, and burning in chest. Must sit up or suffocate; quivering of chin and lower jaw.

Apis 30c: If choking is caused by swollen tongue or throat, e.g., due to allergy, injury, infection, stings, bites, burns.

Carbo Veg 30c: Pale, puffy, bluish face; exhausting sweat and collapse accompanying choking.

Hepar Sulph 30c or Silica 30c: To help dislodge a foreign object.

Note: A sharp object, like a fishbone, can be uncomfortable, but is not as dangerous as an object obstructing the breathing. It is well to check, but often the object passes through, leaving a scratch, which feels sore on swallowing. If a child swallows something smooth without discomfort, take no action. Watch the child's stools for a few days to reassure yourself it has passed through.

SEEK FURTHER ADVICE

- If vomiting or pains in the stomach develop
- If child is wheezing
- If object cannot be dislodged

Cold

A cold is an inflammation of the mucous membranes of the nose and sinus passages caused by a number of viruses. While infections, dampness, drafts, or changes of temperature do not cause a cold, they do weaken resistance to the cold viruses that children come in contact with so easily.

DESCRIPTION

Watery, nasal discharge, blocked nose, sneezing, sore throat, watery eyes, and slight cough. Young children may have a fever as the body tries to throw off the virus. A simple cold usually subsides after a few days.

WHAT TO DO

- Protect child from changes of temperature, dampness, and drafts but do not overdress your child, as this can aggravate the congestion.
- Have child soak in a warm bath to which is added 2 tablespoons of Epsom salts or powdered Ginger to open the pores and help release toxins from the bloodstream.

HERBS

The following can be used as a drink, a gargle, and/or added to bathwater:

As antiseptic: Thyme and Sage
To open the pores and help reduce fever: Lemon Balm
To provide extra nourishment during the cold: Marjoram, Teatree, Thyme, and/or Lavender can also be taken, mixed with honey if desired. (Honey can help healing if not heated above 113°F.
To soothe inflamed area: Coltsfoot
To help build resistance: Regular herbal teas during the win-

ter months also help to ward off the offending viruses. Take Vitamin A- and C-rich herbs such as Mullein, Parsley, Burdock, Rosehip, Comfrey, Yarrow, and Licorice.

HOMEOPATHIC

As homeopathy deals with specific symptoms, please check under the relevant heading (e.g., Cough, Nose—Congestion, Throat). For recurrent colds, or to help prevent a cold during the winter months, see Resistance and Immunity, page 19.

CELL SALTS

Calc Phos: Chronic tendency to take cold.
Calc Sulph: If sore throat is first sign of cold.
Ferr Phos: Fever, dry nose, shivering, child can't get warm.
Kali Mur: If cold develops fully, with blocked nose, white tongue, grayish-white mucous or clear jellylike mucous.
Kali Sulph: Fever with greenish-yellow nasal discharge.
Nat Mur: Watery, nasal discharge, sneezing.

SEE ALSO

Bronchitis, Asthma, or Pneumonia: If noisy breathing or shortness of breath occur.
Cough: If cough becomes worse.
Measles: For runny nose when accompanied by sore throat and red, watery eyes.
Nose: If discharge becomes thick and yellow (may indicate an infection).
Throat and Mumps: If neck glands become swollen or sore.

Cold Sores

A virus (Herpes Simplex) that causes clusters of small fluid-filled blisters to appear, usually on the lips or nostrils. It is often preceded by a burning sensation. The virus can be activated by sunlight or by an upper respiratory tract infection. Also there may be a fever. The sores dry to a scab in 5–10 days.

WHAT TO DO

- Dab Hypercal lotion, Teatree oil, Golden Seal tincture, or Lemon oil directly on to affected area frequently during the day.
- Use diluted Golden Seal tincture to rinse the mouth.
- Apply ice to affected part to help relieve burning sensation.

HERBS

Deficiencies in Calcium and Vitamin D often accompany cold sores, so use Chickweed, Dandelion, Puha, Rosehip, and/or Parsley teas daily, especially if the cold sores often recur.

HOMEOPATHIC

Arsen Alb 30c: Burning, itching, and swelling of the sores. Also use for chronic tendency to cold sores.

Cantharis 30c: For large blisters that smart and burn.

Herpes Simplex Nosode 30c: A dose taken at the end of an attack can help prevent recurrence.

Nat Mur 30c: Fever blisters, eruption around mouth, may be on tongue and under nose.

Rhus Tox 30c: Corners of mouth ulcerate; blisters are angry looking with great itching and tingling.

CELL SALTS

Calc Fluor: Cold sores at corners of mouth.

Nat Mur: Blisters around mouth, cold sores on lip.

Conjunctivitis

The tissue that lines the eyelids and runs out over the eyeball is called the conjunctiva. Inflammation of this tissue, due to cold, irritation, or germ, is called conjunctivitis.

DESCRIPTION

Burning and smarting of the eyelid. When eyelid is pulled away from eye lightly, the normally pink lid appears reddened. Tears may flood out although the child is not crying, and there is often sensitivity to light. There may be a yellow discharge, especially evident upon waking with gummed eyes.

WHAT TO DO

Make a solution of Hypercal and/or Euphrasia tincture (5 drops to half-glass of water). Moisten cotton balls with solution and use to rub away discharge. Sweep from inner to outer edge of the eye and be sure to use a new cotton ball for each sweep. When eye is clear, place 2 drops of same solution into infected eye. Place the drops carefully into inner corner of eye. Repeat eyedrops 3 times daily for 3–4 days.

HERBS

Use a weak solution of these herbs to bathe the eyes: Eyebright, Chamomile, and/or Golden Seal. The same mixture can be taken as a tea.

HOMEOPATHIC

Arsen Alb 30c: Intense sensitivity to light with heat and burning in eyes.

Belladonna 30c: Sudden, violent symptoms; swollen, staring, brilliant dilated eyes that are worse from exposure to heat and daylight. Eyes red, feel full of sand, better from rubbing.

Euphrasia 30c: Lids stuck together after sleep, constant thick, painful discharge with inclination to blink. Eyelids red and swollen. Tears scald and irritate cheeks.

Mercurius 30c: Profuse discharge that burns the cheeks; extreme intolerance of light.

Pulsatilla 30c: Yellow bland discharge; itchy, sore lids.

CELL SALTS

Ferr Phos: First stage of inflammation.

Kali Sulph: Yellow-green colored crusts on lids.

Nat Phos: Discharge of yellow matter; eyelids stick together in morning.

Constipation

Retarded bowel action, causing either total absence or difficulty in the passage of feces (stools).

Poor bowel habits begin in childhood. If the bowels do not move regularly (daily), the kidney, skin, liver, lungs, and lymph have to work harder and eventually other health problems are created.

WHAT TO DO

Commercial laxatives can irritate the bowel, force peristaltic action, and tire the bowel muscle.

- *Drink adequate fluids:* As a rule, find child's weight in kilograms, and give this amount of fluid ounces daily. To each glass of water can be added 1 drop of Rosemary oil.
- Exercise regularly.
- Increase dietary fiber with whole-grain breads and muesli.
- Fresh Vegetables: Fresh beans, beetroot (top included), carrots, celery, lettuce, and cucumber.
- Fruits: Figs, prunes, pears, peaches, grapes, berries, pineapple.
- Eliminate junk foods, white flour, sugar products, and cheese.

- On rising drink a glass of water that has the juice from half a lemon added to it.
- Cold-pressed Olive oil (1 tsp.–1 Tbsp.) should be included in the daily diet.
- Make homemade jelly using agar instead of gelatin (2Tbsp agar to 2.1 cups of boiling water; half boiling water, half fruit juice; or Rosehip tea). Flavor with honey or lemon juice. Served with fruit, this is easily taken by a child and helps to loosen the bowel movements. Can be taken daily.

HERBS

Licorice, Rosemary, Linseed, Oatstraw, Borage, and Senna. (When using Senna, always add a pinch of Ginger to alleviate the gripping pains that Senna can cause. Do not use Senna for babies.)

HOMEOPATHIC

Apis 30c: Shooting upward pains in rectum before or during bowel movement; often passes stool while urinating.

Bryonia 30c: Stools are dry, hard, large, and difficult to pass.

Causticum 30c: Unsuccessful desire with pain and great straining. Easier to pass stool by standing. Nat Mur 30c: Dry, crumbling stool, difficult to expel with bleeding and pain in rectum.

Nux Vomica 30c: Frequent, ineffectual urging, worse after party or overeating.

Psorinum 200c: For stubborn cases that do not respond to above remedies.

CELL SALTS

Calc Fluor: Weak rectal muscles. Huge accumulation with anal cracks, very painful piles, great difficulty in expelling waste matter.

Ferr Phos: Constipation with inflammation, heat or pain, and piles.

Kali Sulph: Constipation with yellow, slimy tongue.

Nat Mur: Constipation with headache, maybe hemorrhoids or sore feeling in anus after passing stool; dry stools difficult to pass.

Nat Phos: Alternates with diarrhea, all efforts result in nothing.

Nat Sulph: Hard, knotty stools.

Silica: For pale children, bowel movement never seems completed.

Cough

Reflex expulsive action to remove foreign bodies or mucous from the breathing passages.

WHAT TO DO

For foreign objects, see Choking. Coughs usually go with a cold but can also herald more serious illness.

HERBS

Soothe the breathing passages with Marshmallow, Licorice, or Coltsfoot. Strengthen the lungs against invading germs with Mullein, Hyssop, Comfrey, or Teatree.

The cough may become looser at first; this is a sign of mucous loosening and being expelled. It should be encouraged, not suppressed.

HOMEOPATHIC

The cough remedies are very specific to the individual case. We mention here only those remedies cited in our health kit. Further remedies can be found in the recommended homeopathic books.

Aconite 30c: Worse for exposure to dry, cold weather; also worse from entering a warm room; short of breath, short, dry barking cough, which wakes child from sleep. Little or no expectoration.

Antim Tart 30c: Whistling or rattling mucous with little expectoration; maybe pain in chest, drowsy and sweaty; must sit up to cough.

Arsen Alb 30c: Frequent sneezing, chilly, dry hacking cough with no expectoration; better if head is kept warm. Worse after midnight.

Bacillinum 30c: Lingering, stubborn, or recurring coughs worse at night and early morning; recurring after antibiotics.

Belladonna 30c: Moaning and crying; burning, throbbing; tickling cough with blood-streaked mucous.

Bryonia 30c: Hard, hollow, very painful cough with raw throat and hoarse voice. Worse from eating and from warm room. Must hold chest during cough.

Gelsemium 30c: Summer colds and influenza-related coughs; sneezing and fullness at root of nose with headache, heavy eyes, maybe general aches.

Hepar Sulph 30c: Bouts of dry, hoarse, suffocative coughs. Child is sensitive to touch, pain, drafts, and cold, dry air. Almost chokes on the phlegm.

Lycopodium 30c: Deep, hollow, tickling cough. Worse 4–8 P.M.

Nux Vomica 30c: Painful, spasmodic cough. Gagging and retching with bursting headache. Feels cold and likes to be covered.

Phosphorus 30c: Persistent cough affecting the throat; worse from talking and going from warm to cold air.

Pulsatilla 30c: Persistent cough that is dry in the evening and loose in the morning; better in the open air, some thick, frothy mucous.

CELL SALTS

Calc Phos: Suffocating cough, better lying down. Any mucous is like raw egg white.

Ferr Phos: Will often cut short an attack that begins with a short, dry, tickling cough with no expectoration.

Kali Mur: Hoarse, croupy-sounding cough with white tongue and mucous.

Kali Sulph: Rattly cough with yellow, shiny mucous, worse in a warm room and evening; better in cool, open air.

Mag Phos: Cough sounds like whooping cough but with no discharge of mucous.

Nat Mur: Clear, watery, salty discharge, which may come from eyes, nose or mouth, always accompanies cough.

Nat Sulph: Thick yellow-green mucous, worse in damp weather; pain in chest on coughing.

Silica: Thick, yellow-green mucous, worse from cold drinks and in the morning.

TYPES OF COUGH

Coughs can also indicate a more serious complaint; it is well to check the symptoms below and, where necessary, refer to the relevant page.

Asthma: Wheeze from deep in lungs, difficulty in expelling air, pounding in chest.

Bronchitis: May start as a cold but moves to the chest with rattly cough, feeling of tightness, maybe a slight temperature rise, yellow mucous may be coughed up.

Cold: Cough not severe, no shortness of breath or noisy breathing.

Croup: Loud, barking cough, noisy on breathing in, hoarse voice, shortness of breath.

Measles: The measles cough usually comes when other measles symptoms have developed.

Pneumonia: Very ill; rapid breathing, high temperature accompany cough.

Whooping Cough: Spasms of coughs in rapid succession; child cannot draw breath until spasm is over; this desperate sucking in of air causes the characteristic "whoop."

Cramp

Violent muscle spasm in one or more muscles brought on by interference with circulation to the part.

Cramp is caused by one of the following: overuse; excessive jarring or tearing of muscles; poor circulation, resulting in inability to deliver essential nutrients (especially Calcium, Magnesium, and Vitamins) to the body. This is especially common during pregnancy.

DESCRIPTION

Muscle knots and shortens, causing sharp, grabbing pain and stiffness. Muscle cannot be used during spasm. Cramps are often worse in the afternoon, in hot weather, or during sleep.

With internal cramps (e.g., chest or stomach) there can be breathlessness, night sweats, dizziness, or weakness.

WHAT TO DO

- Gentle stretching.
- Light feather touch to affected part.
- Alternate hot and cold packs (hot water bottle or hot flannel and ice-filled flannel), always ending with a cold pack.

For recurring cramps: Avoid low-calcium foods like meat, liver, wheat, and citrus (which robs the body of calcium); eat more millet, sesame seed, yogurt, oats, milk, alfalfa sprouts.

If cramps are a result of salt loss: Replace by drinking flat soda or electrolyte solution as a temporary measure (2.1 cups boiled water, 8 tsp. sugar, $\frac{1}{2}$ tsp. salt). However, it is more important to correct the mineral imbalance (see below).

HERBS

Recurrent problems indicate a mineral imbalance, so drink herbs rich in Calcium, Magnesium, and Vitamins C and E: Valerian,

Dandelion, Comfrey, Thyme, Chamomile, Yellow Dock, and Sage

Stomach Cramps: Use one or more of the following: Peppermint, Chamomile, Fennel Seed, Catnip, and/or ground Cloves. Apply a few drops of Teatree oil externally to the affected area.

HOMEOPATHIC

Calc Carb 30c: Helps to remove a tendency to cramps.

Cocculus 30c: Cramps in chest.

Colocynth 30c: Cramp in hip or stomach, causing child to bend double.

Cupric 30c: For cramps in calves, soles, and palms.

Lycopodium 30c: Cramps in toes, calves, and fingers.

CELL SALTS

Calc phos: If cramps occur during teething.

Mag Phos: Main remedy for sudden cramps.

Croup

Juvenile form of laryngitis, usually caused by a virus creating an infection in the larynx region.

DESCRIPTION

Starts as a mild upper respiratory infection, with some hoarseness. Then child wakes at night, clutches at throat with difficult breathing, husky voice, and characteristic dry, barking cough. This lasts half an hour to three hours and then suddenly eases. Croup is very rare under six months and usually occurs between the ages of two and four.

WHAT TO DO

Croup without a fever: Treat by filling the room with steam (boil kettle or run hot tap in bathroom). Reassure and stay with child. A few drops of Teatree, Eucalyptus, and/or Lavender oil may be added to steaming water. Check breathing 2–3 hours after attack. Keep the room warm for the next few nights.

Croup with a fever: This is more serious as it is accompanied by a chest cold. Breathing difficulty comes on more slowly but can come any time; steaming only partly relieves.

HERBS

Give frequent sips of hot Lemon/Mint drinks, sweetened with honey if necessary; give child a bath to which has been added 2 tsp. Ginger powder or 2 tsp. baking soda.

Sip frequently a warm herb drink made from any or all of the following: Lemon, Thyme, Mullein, Catnip, and/or Garlic. Add one drop of Lobelia tincture for each year of the child's life (some children react strongly if larger amounts are given). These herbs help to soothe and calm the breathing passages and help fight any infection.

HOMEOPATHIC

A common approach is to alternate Aconite, Hepar Sulph, and Spongia at 15–minute intervals until relief is obtained.

Aconite 30c: Child is restless and anxious; after exposure to cold dry winds, cough becomes hard, dry, and barking.

Hepar Sulph 30c: Chilly and sweaty; loose rattling cough; worse from least uncovering.

Spongia 30c: Noisy, rasping tight cough without wheeze or rattle; maybe tough phlegm difficult to cough up and usually swallowed; breathing is harsh.

Note: If throat is swollen so that child is choking and lips have a blue tinge, give Apis 30c at 15–minute intervals for three doses (check Diphtheria) and seek medical advice.

CELL SALTS

Alternate Ferr Phos and Kali Mur. Add the following, if necessary:
Calc Sulph: If croup is recurrent. Take regularly for several
weeks.
Mag Phos: Great difficulty in breathing.

SEEK MEDICAL ADVICE

- If, when child breathes in, the abdominal wall draws in more than a little. This means there is considerable lung obstruction.
- If noisy breathing persists, or if child becomes blue, restless, and struggles very hard to breathe. (This child would need hospitalization.)

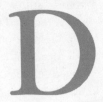

Diabetes—Juvenile

A blood sugar problem caused by a defect in the pancreas that results in a deficiency of insulin in the body. Insulin is involved in the metabolism of sugars and a deficiency causes an excess of sugar in the blood. This disorder may be inherited or be a result of a pancreatic disease.

Complications: Infections, unconsciousness, eye problems, renal failure, arteriosclerosis, glomerulosclerosis, proteinuria, gangrene of the feet. Pregnancy complications in later life.

DESCRIPTION

General weakness, irritability, weight loss, hunger, thirst, excessive flow of urine, bed-wetting. Can cause loss of consciousness (coma).

Urine tests immediately after a meal show excess sugar levels in the blood.

WHAT TO DO

We advise that you seek the help of an experienced natural health practitioner for this illness, as correctly used natural remedies can offer significant help for diabetes. But we also advise that you keep in touch with a medical practitioner to monitor progress.

Many juvenile diabetes cases can be controlled by diet alone. However, in all cases it is important to set up an eating pattern that avoids peaks of glucose entering the blood. Each diet must be tailor-made to the individual concerned, so seek dietary advice from a naturopath or dietitian. Keep in mind that slow release of blood sugar is required throughout the day, so whole-grain carbohydrates and proteins should be eaten—preferably in the form of four to six small meals rather than three large ones.

Avoid refined carbohydrates such as sugar and white flour products.

Certain foods are considered to be helpful for insulin production: barley, cabbage, lettuce, banana, oats, olives, papaya, turnips, sweet potato, bitter gourd.

HERBS

To help regulate blood sugar: Burdock, Wild Carrot, Nettle, Oats, Wormwood, Juniper, Garlic. Bitter gourd (Karela) is highly recommended. Tumeric, taken medicinally (2–3 times daily) as a powder, $1/4$ tsp. mixed with herb tea or Aloe Vera juice.

HOMEOPATHIC

Arsen Alb 30c: Great weakness, hunger, and thirst; dry mouth, excessive urination.

Bryonia 30c: Dry lips, persistent bitter taste, morose, dispirited, loses strength through inability to eat. Thirst for large drinks.

Insulin 3x: A homeopathic way to take insulin. Should be taken under the guidance of a homeopath.

Lactic Acid 30c: Profuse urine, light yellow glucose in urine; nausea, debility, voracious appetite; constipation; dry skin and tongue.

Phos Acid 30c: Nervous, worse from grief, worry, or anxiety; indifference, apathy, great debility; bruised feeling in muscles; loss of appetite, unquenchable thirst; sugary, jellylike or milky urine.

Plumbum 30c: Great hunger, sweet taste in mouth, sweetish belching and vomiting; obstinate constipation.

CELL SALTS

Nat Sulph and Nat Phos: Chief remedies. Take daily as they

help to stimulate the pancreatic secretions and therefore help the functions of this organ. Also help to eliminate waste fluids from the body.

Calc Phos: For weak thirsty, restless children worse from depressing emotions. Bed wetting when associated with general weakness or debility.

Nat Mur: Great wasting of energy; excessive flow of urine with thirst and constipation.

Kali Phos: Nervous weakness; voracious hunger; sleeplessness, coma; bed wetting when associated with nervous weakness.

SEEK MEDICAL ADVICE

Most children with diabetes need insulin injections and quickly become expert at managing this for themselves.

Diaper Rash

Seen as sore, red, scalded skin on bottom and diaper area.

WHAT TO DO

HERBS

Any of the following may be helpful when applied locally to the rash: Calendula ointment, Apricot Kernel or Avocado oil, Aloe Vera gel.

HOMEOPATHIC

Borax 30c: Rash between thighs in babies subject to thrush.

Calc Carb 30c: In babies who perspire easily with cold hands and feet; eruptions may be pustular or scaly-looking; itching, smarting, worse from cold.

Graphites 30c: Skin harsh, dry, thickened, rough and easily

chafed. Better from warmth and dryness. Usually accompanied by constipation.

Hepar Sulph 30c: Genital area inflamed and itching; very sensitive when exposed to cold air, touch, undressing. Better from warmth.

Sulphur 30c: Dry, itchy, scaly, red eruption on genital area. Worse at night, and in bed.

WHAT TO DO—EXTERNAL APPLICATIONS

Urtica Urens cream or tincture (10 drops to half-glass water).

CELL SALTS

Nat Phos counteracts too much acidity.

Nat Mur: For chafed skin.

Crush three tablets of either cell salt, mix with 1 Tbs. water and apply to the rash.

Rinse diapers thoroughly in 1 Tbs. vinegar per 2 cup of water. Be aware that, in some cases, disposable diapers can aggravate diaper rash. Expose skin to air a few hours every day. Do not leave wet diapers on.

Long-continuing or *severe diaper rash* may be an indication of a more serious skin condition, such as eczema or psoriasis.

Diarrhea

Occurs when the normal rate of movement of waste matter through the digestive tract is sped up or if absorption in the bowels is inhibited by disease; the contents will still be liquid when they reach the rectum and so loose movements result. Three or more loose movements a day is considered to be diarrhea.

Acute diarrhea can be caused by infections either in the gut or outside the gut (e.g., tonsillitis, ear infections, urinary infections);

anxiety or fear; irritants taken into the stomach and bowel via food; laxatives; metabolic disturbance, e.g., nutritional deficiency, allergic reactions, weakened digestive organs; antibiotic treatment; unripe, or greasy foods. The poorly nourished child is the most prone to diarrhea.

Chronic diarrhea is the result of bowel disease and must be treated by a competent naturopath, homeopath, or medical doctor.

WHAT TO DO

1. Take no foods for twenty-four hours.
2. Alternate hot and cold compresses to abdomen if painful (use hot flannel or hot water bottle, and ice wrapped in flannel).
3. Take plenty of fluids. *It is important to guard against dehydration caused by excessive fluid loss through the bowel.* Any or all of the following can be taken throughout the day:

   - Water with oil of Clove or Rosemary (1 drop only of each to a cup of water)
   - Chamomile Tea
   - Cold Black Tea
   - Electrolyte Solution (2.1 cups boiled water, 8 tsp. sugar, ½ tsp. salt)
   - Kaolin-Pectin mixture: Stocked by pharmacists. Prevents absorption of bacterial toxins by forming a film on the intestinal wall. Also absorbs some of the toxins. The nutrients are quickly firmed up and temporary relief is provided. However, it is still wise to provide nutritional fluids wherever possible.

When camping or away from home, cool, flat (made flat by heating) soda is useful and readily available.

If breastfeeding, continue and add fluid drinks as directed for mother and/or baby.

4. Sustaining drinks:

   Vegetable drink: Cut 2–5 vegetables into small pieces and bring to the boil in enough water to leave 2– 3 cups of juice. Simmer for 20–30 minutes. This can be taken warm or cold throughout the day and supplies adequate vitamins and minerals. Best vegetables are potato (just thickly peeled skins), parsnip, kumara/sweet potato, parsley.

   Fruit drink: Blend organic apples in blender for apple sauce, or cut up apples (pips and skins included) and boil in enough water to leave 2–3 cups of juice. Pulp can be kept as a first solid after 24–hour fast is complete.

   Grain drink: Simmer 60 gms. barley, rice, or oatmeal in 2.1 cups of water for 30 minutes, then strain.

5. First foods—If your child is distressingly hungry and dissatisfied with fluids, give grated raw apple including pips (no other raw fruit should be taken) for the older child every two hours. For the younger child, make a Slippery Elm porridge and mix with any or all of the following: stewed apple, bananas, ginger, carob, cinnamon or nutmeg (until bowels firm up). Dry crackers or rice may also be useful for the older child.

HERBS

As antiseptic against bacteria: Golden Seal.
For stomach pains: Calendula, Catnip, Fennel Seed,
    Peppermint, or Slippery Elm.
To help tonify the system: Gentian or Rhubarb Root, Comfrey.
Take with meals: 1 drop of Clove or Rosemary essential oil
    in water.

HOMEOPATHIC

Arsen Alb 30c: Diarrhea may be caused by spoiled foods or
    too much fruit. Frequent scanty, offensive stools that burn
    the skin. Great exhaustion follows stools.

Calc Phos 30c: Green, slimy, undigested stools, worse during teething. Noisy, spluttering stools.

China 30c: Debilitating, involuntary, painless, diarrhea with putrid smell. Worse after eating fruit.

Colocynth 30c: Diarrhea with colic, better from bending double. Worse from slightest food or drink.

Gelsemium 30c: Diarrhea yellow and changeable, brought on by nerves, fright, or excitement.

Hepar Sulph 30c: Clay-colored, sour-smelling stools.

Mercurius 30c: Slimy, bloody stools. Never-get-done feeling.

Podophyllum 30c: Morning stool, painless watery yellow and profuse and gushing. Worse after eating and drinking. Maybe a natural stool later in day.

Rhus Tox 30c: If recurring problem. May have no appetite. May be worse from apple juice.

CELL SALTS

Calc Phos: If diarrhea occurs during teething.

Ferr Phos: Undigested stools come on suddenly with fever.

Kali Mur: Pale-colored stools, worse from rich foods.

Kali Phos: Foul-smelling diarrhea.

Kali Sulph: Yellow stools and cramps.

LONG-TERM APPROACH

Cut down on dairy products, white flour products, meat, salt, and pepper. Be sure to include plenty of natural yogurt to replace friendly bacteria to the intestines. Check the cleanliness of the household. Protect food from flies. Wash hands. Wash baby bottles, etc., thoroughly. Check at medical laboratory for intestinal parasites. There are homeopathic Nosodes to act against these. Seek homeopathic advice.

SEEK MEDICAL AID

- If child shows signs of dehydration: i.e., skin does not rebound on pinching lightly.

- If child appears limp, pale, and unaware of surroundings.
- If child has bloody stool.

Digestive Problems

Stomach ache, nausea, heartburn, colic, indigestion, gastroenteritis, vomiting.

DESCRIPTION

Poor digestion and stomach problems occur through faulty eating habits, poor spinal alignment, overtiredness, stress, poor living habits, illness picked up while traveling. Acute irritation can also be caused by infectious illness, bacterial infection (e.g., food poisoning or staphylococcal infection), scarlet fever, pneumonia, viral infections (e.g., measles, hepatitis, influenza), and allergies, e.g., to shellfish. During a digestive disturbance the natural reaction of the body is to remove the food as quickly as possible; therefore vomiting often results. Otherwise, the food may begin to ferment in the stomach, causing heartburn and nausea, progressing to colic, pain, or swelling in the abdomen. The final result may be diarrhea or constipation.

See also: Allergy, Appendicitis, Diarrhea, Constipation, Poisoning.

WHAT TO DO

- Do not give child any food.
- Over twenty-four hours give fluids only. Fresh unsweetened fruit or vegetable juices can be given (best are lemon, carrot, apple, and pineapple).
- Alternate hot and cold packs (hot water bottle for five minutes, ice pack for two minutes) on abdomen and continue with the one that gives more relief. A washcloth soaked in warm Castor oil can be very soothing.
- After acute symptoms subside, give (for two days) a light diet only consisting of fruit, vegetables, and homemade soup.

- Gradually return to normal diet, watching for any reactions to specific foods. These may cause a recurrence of the problem or indicate an allergy (see Allergy).
- For pain after meals: 1 tsp. Cider vinegar to a glass of warm water and honey. Can be taken first thing in the morning and half an hour before meals if desired, to aid digestion.
- Slippery Elm Powder: 1 tsp. mixed with yogurt before food eases the whole digestive tract. Papaya is also very soothing to the stomach.
- Never give cold milk if your child is prone to digestive problems. Always heat milk first and add a pinch of digestive-aiding spice such as Cardamom, Ginger, or Fennel.

HERBS

Drink a tea made from one or more of the following herbs, or add to a mild food like Slippery Elm (see above).

Pain, flatulence, heartburn, colic, cramp: Irish Moss, Meadowsweet, Aniseed, Peppermint, Cloves, Ginger, Nutmeg, Parsley, Dill, Fennel, Comfrey, and Chickweed.

Anxiety felt in the stomach, and difficulty swallowing food: Valerian, Skullcap, Chamomile, Lavender and/or Rosemary.

"Sore tummies" often worse from nerves (e.g., in the morning before school): Take herbs for anxiety and pain as above. Bach Flower Remedies deal specifically with emotions and are very helpful in these situations. See your health shop for Bach Flower Remedies and books about them.

Nausea and vomiting (gastroenteritis): Clove, Peppermint, Basil, Cinnamon, and/or Dill.

To help soothe the irritated digestive tract, especially after vomiting: Comfrey, Slippery Elm, Yarrow, Golden Seal, and/or Licorice.

Poor appetite, and as a tonic after digestive disturbance: Meadowsweet, Gentian, Licorice, Couchgrass, and/or Peppermint.

HOMEOPATHIC

Antim Tart 30c: For nausea, retching, vomiting, colic, thirst for small cold drinks, better from belching; craves acids or apples.

Arsen Alb 30c: Severe vomiting; burning gripping pain with heavy feeling in stomach. May be from food poisoning.

Bryonia 30c: Acidity, weight and fullness in stomach, nausea and faintness when sitting up.

Carbo Veg 30c: Flatulence, stomach pain extending up to chest or back; food poisoning from bad fish or meat; deathly cold but feels hot inside; worse from ice cream, better from belching.

Ipecac 30c: Intense nausea and vomiting with sleepiness. Clean tongue.

Kali Bich 30c: Nausea, bitter vomiting, cutting pain soon after eating. Worse from meat.

Lycopodium 30c: Dilated stomach, feeling of fullness and heaviness immediately after eating. Child desires sweets.

Nux Vomica 30c: Nausea; empty retching, white coating on back of tongue. Irritable and cranky. Worse from overeating and worse in morning. A feeling of "if only I could vomit."

Pulsatilla 30c: Vomiting, may be caused by rich food, cream, etc. Thickly coated white tongue. Weight in stomach an hour or two after eating. Much wind, belching, and heartburn with dry mouth and foul taste. Worse morning.

CELL SALTS

Calc Phos: Abnormal appetite, craves bacon, ham, and salty food. Gaseous belching, colic in babies, vomiting with teething.

Kali Mur: Loss of appetite, tender abdomen. Grayish-white coating on tongue.

Kali Phos: Child will often complain of heartburn or sore heart; worse from emotional stress.

Kali Sulph: Pain in stomach, worse from anything tight. Yellow coating on tongue.

Mag Phos: Vomiting and diarrhea, spasmodic pains and cramps, burning sensation, nausea, hiccups. Child craves sweets.

Nat Mur: Vomiting of sour fluid, not food. Bad breath, very thirsty, dislike of bread. Helps secretion of hydrochloric acid in stomach.

Nat Phos: Acidity and painful belching, worse from fat food and eating, vomiting of curdled milk; nausea. Helps destroy intestinal worms.

Silica: Child vomits as soon as it nurses; disgust for warm food; hunger and chilliness.

SEEK MEDICAL ADVICE

- If pain remains for more than four hours, or if you suspect appendicitis.
- If bowel movements are dark red, jellylike texture.
- If swelling develops in groin with abdominal pain and vomiting.
- For food poisoning.

Diphtheria

THIS DISEASE MUST BE REPORTED TO YOUR DOCTOR OR YOUR LOCAL HEALTH DEPARTMENT.

A contagious infection of the throat, nose, or larynx that can be fatal and which causes serious effects on other parts of the body. (Fortunately, it is no longer common.)

DESCRIPTION

Sore throat involving tonsils and larynx; mild fever and general sick feeling; throat membrane has glistening yellow-gray appearance that bleeds if wiped; foul-smelling breath; breathing can be tight and difficult with hoarseness and a hacking cough.

Most common season: winter and autumn. Incubation period: 3–4 days only.

Isolation period: For two weeks from date of onset until cultures from nose and throat fail to show presence of the infection.

Recovery time: May be up to six months.

Complications: Can affect the heart, lungs, and nervous system, so ensure that expert advice is sought immediately.

SEEK MEDICAL ADVICE IMMEDIATELY

The following procedure is included for your information and can be helpful in restoring to full health after medical treatment or until medical aid arrives.

WHAT TO DO

Reduce diet to fresh fruit juices, vegetable juices, and soups. Papaya or papain enzyme helps to dissolve membrane.

HERBS

Make a mixture from the following:

To cleanse: Horehound or Sage.
To soothe inflamed throat: Slippery Elm and/or Marshmallow.
To provide extra nourishment: Lemon juice, rind.
To purify blood: Golden Seal and/or Echinacea.

Inhalation: Oils of Lemon and Eucalyptus can be used as an inhalation (2–3 drops into steaming water) to breathe, or gargle (1–2 drops with glass of water).

HOMEOPATHIC

After suspected contact: see Resistance and Immunity, page 19.

Baptisia 30c: General sick feeling, difficult breathing, pressure at root of nose, with confused feeling in head. Can only swallow liquids.

Fachesis 30c: Blackish throat membrane, worse from swallowing and pressure. Feeling of strangulation.

Gelsemium 30c: Very difficult swallowing, paralyzed feeling in throat, putrid breath, heavy dull headache.

Kali Bich 30c: Pain extends to neck and shoulders; swollen glands, tongue is dry and red, or has yellow coating.

Merc Cyanatus 30c: Fetid breath, grayish mouth membranes, ulcerations in mouth, hoarseness and pain from talking, nausea, biliousness, terrible headache.

Diphtherinum 200c (Nosode—see page 21): To help clear a severe case or for lingering aftereffects of the disease. *Do not give while disease is incubating.*

CELL SALTS

Nat Phos, Ferr Phos and Kali Mur can be given together every two hours at the first sign of fever, illness, and sore throat.

Kali Phos: For exhaustion and offensive breath.

Kali Mur and Calc Phos: Alternate for difficult breathing.

TO BUILD RESISTANCE

To help strengthen the immune system and restore to full health after the disease or vaccination, see Resistance and Immunity, page 19.

E

Ear

1 Glue Ear
2 Hearing
3 Middle Ear Infection
4 Outer Ear Infection
5 Object in Ear
6 Wax in Ears

1 Glue Ear

An accumulation of thick mucous in the middle ear. Hearing is lessened, child often talks more loudly than usual. There is usually no pain.

Glue ear in and of itself is not necessarily a problem, but it can make ear infections more likely. Time may eventually clear the narrow passages, but any hearing loss must be carefully checked and treated.

WHAT TO DO

HERBS

To help break down mucous in any part of the body: Comfrey, Bayberry, Queens Delight, Fenugreek, Golden Seat, Elecampane, and Coltsfoot.

Calc Carb 30c: Difficult hearing with cracking noises in ear and full feeling.

Kali Mur 30c: For catarrhal conditions of the middle ear where child hears cracking noises and ear feels congested on swallowing or blowing nose.

Kali Sulph 30c: Deafness with discharge of yellow matter.

Merc Dulcis 30c: Blocked Eustachian tube, offensive breath; difficult hearing, worse during a cold.

Pulsatilla 30c: Difficult hearing as if ear were stuffed. Maybe some thick, bland discharge.

Other remedies are best chosen by a competent homeopath, so seek advice if none of the above remedies are suitable.

CELL SALTS

Alternate Ferr Phos and Kali Mur for deafness following a cold.

Calc Sulph: For difficult hearing with thick, yellow discharge.

2 Hearing

If a child does not respond to quiet, unexpected noises by six months, if there is little babbling by one year, or if there is any doubt in your mind about your child's hearing ability, a proper hearing test is appropriate. These are available either through your family medical doctor or health care company.

A competent homeopath may be able to provide some assistance with this problem. Success with homeopathic remedies largely depends on the cause of the hearing difficulty.

On the inside of the eardrum, the middle ear must stay full of air to transmit sounds efficiently from the eardrum to the hearing nerve. When fluid fills this space, caused by a blockage in the tube leading to the nose, tone and hearing are lessened. If this space is constantly fluid-filled, a "glue ear" develops, and if bacteria invade this area, an ear infection develops.

3 Middle Ear Infection

Child is sick, irritable, has earache, and usually tugs on ear. Partial hearing loss. Red and angry-looking eardrum. Usually associated with a cold, as nasal blockage causes middle eardrum to fill with fluid. It can also accompany measles or bronchitis, or be caused by excessive swimming.

An ear infection that is left alone will either clear by a reopening of the nasal passages or by perforation of the eardrum, causing a gooey, yellow-white fluid to flow out of the ear. This perforation will almost always heal by itself, but if it happens several times, there can be scarring on the eardrum, which lessens hearing ability. It is therefore important that each infection be completely cleared to help prevent repeated infections and hearing damage.

Complications of an untreated ear infection can in some cases be mastoiditis or meningitis.

WHAT TO DO—ACUTE EAR INFECTION

Have your local ear clinic or medical doctor monitor the state of the eardrum during the infection.

HERBS

To help ease the pain: Lobelia tincture (1 drop for every year of child's age—5 drops maximum). Some children react strongly to this herb, so it is wise to use a low dose. Give on a teaspoon with water internally at 15–minute intervals. Further pain relief may be obtained with 1 drop of Mullein oil or Lemon oil placed on a warm teaspoon with 10–20 drops of pure Olive oil and poured into the ear duct. If there are signs of perforated eardrum, intense pain, or discharge from the ear, do not put anything into the ear.

To calm and induce sleep: Elder and Chamomile.

To help purify blood and cleanse the ear canal: Golden Seal and Queens Delight.

HOMEOPATHIC

Aconite 30c: For acute onset in an otherwise healthy child. Redness and pain better from hot applications. Very thirsty.

Belladonna 30c: Sudden and throbbing pain, with red, hot face worse from least jar or knock.

Chamomilla 30c: Child is angry, cross, and wants to be carried. Worse from heat. Cannot tolerate pain. One cheek red, the other pale.

Hepar Sulph 30c: Hot, maybe itching ear with sore throat, pus discharge, worse in a draft, sensitive to touch.

Kali Bich 30c: Tearing pains or sharp stitches in ears following congestion in nose and throat.

Mercurius 30c: Discharge can be thick or thin, but always streaked with blood; boils in external canal, worse from warmth of bed.

Merc Dulcis 30c: Blocked Eustachian tube, infection with offensive breath and difficult hearing.

Pulsatilla 30c: Ear feels stuffed, sharp pulsating pains, discharge is thick and bland, better in the open air, worse in a warm room, and at night.

CELL SALTS

Calc Phos: Earache with swelling of glands about the ear and maybe a clear discharge.

Ferr Phos: For throbbing, burning pain; external ear may be red and hot.

Kali Mur: Swollen glands and Eustachian tubes; noises in ears on blowing nose.

Kali Sulph: Earache with thin, yellow discharge, yellow coating on tongue and sharp pains.

Mag Phos: Earache with sharp, shooting pains.

WHAT TO DO—LONG-TERM TREATMENT

- If infections are not completely cleared they will recur.
- Check for food allergy, especially dairy products (see Allergy).

For incomplete return to health after infectious diseases such as mumps, see page 19 (Resistance).

HERBS

Drink herbs daily to detoxify the ear canal: Queens Delight, Elecampane or Burdock
As an antiseptic: Golden Seal
To help loosen and move the mucous: Comfrey or Fenugreek

These herbs will need to be continued for at least three weeks.

HOMEOPATHIC

Calc Carb 30c: Chronic enlarged glands, pressing, throbbing, cracking noises, worse from slightest cold about neck and ears.
Causticum 30c: Wax, middle ear catarrh, blocked feeling. Roaring rushing noises or reechoing of sounds in ears.
Medorrhinum 30c: Pains and deafness associated with chronic catarrhal conditions in children. Parotidinum 30c: If ear problems have lingered since child had mumps.
Streptococcin 30c: Constantly recurring infections with history of streptococcal infection.

CELL SALTS

As for Acute Infection. Also Calc Sulph: If there is a thick, yellow or bloody discharge.

4 Outer Ear Infection

Infection of the skin lining, eardrum, or outer ear canal. Causes pain, itching, and discharge from the ear, often with reduced hearing because the ear canal is blocked.

Don't use cotton swabs to penetrate the ear canal, as the wax lining will protect the skin surface and absorb germs and bacteria, thereby preventing fungal growth. The blockage will clear itself during the healing process.

HOMEOPATHIC

Belladonna 30c: Red, swollen and painful to touch.
Calc Carb 30c: Eruption on and behind ear; enlarged glands.
Causticum 30c: Helps to break down accumulated wax.
Graphites 30c: Moisture and eruption behind ears.
Hepar Sulph 30c: Itching in ears, pus discharge.
Mezereum 30c: Ears feel too much open as of a cold wind; likes to bore fingers into ears.
Pulsatilla 30c: External ear is swollen and red.

5 Object in Ear

If eardrum is NOT perforated, flood ear with tepid water (signs of perforation: intense pain and discharge—may have feeling as of a hole in ear); have child tip head so that water flows upward, not toward the drum. If this does not dislodge the object, seek further advice.

Insects can often be floated out with warm Olive oil (temperature: just hot enough so that spoon with oil feels comfortable against your own upper lip).
Give Aconite 30c if needed for agitation.
Give Arnica 30c two doses before and two doses after any surgical treatment.

6 Wax in Ears

Do not attempt to clear wax during an infection.
Use a teaspoon of warm Olive oil (temperature: just hot enough so the spoon with oil feels comfortable against your own upper lip).

Have child place his/her head on pillow with affected ear up, pull earlobe up and back, and pour Olive oil in gently until canal is full. Press firmly on mound in front of ear. Pumping action forces the oil in between the wax. Have child remain in this position for ten minutes, then allow oil to drain out.

HOMEOPATHIC

Causticum 30c: To break down accumulation of ear wax.

Eczema

Starts as itchy, red skin; may weep clear fluid after it is scratched. This forms crusts when it dries. If untreated, the skin becomes less red, dry, and thickened. Often it starts on cheeks or forehead in babies; bends of knees or elbows in toddlers. It is not contagious.

Causes can be any of the following:

- Sensitivity or allergy to something contacted or eaten.
- Faulty metabolism, constipation, poor elimination of toxins.
- Nutritional deficiencies.

WHAT TO DO—INTERNAL APPLICATIONS

We advise that you seek the help of an experienced natural health practitioner. Natural remedies can offer significant help to eczema sufferers. Determine irritating agent, see Allergy.

- Treat emotional aspects with Bach Flowers—a stressful situation can be sufficient to trigger a recurrence of eczema. (Books on Bach Flower Remedies are available at most health shops.)
- Good foods to eat: avocado, dandelion, melons, sunflower seeds, and goat's milk.

- Check for presence of Candida Albicans (see Thrush, p. 213, for more information).

WHAT TO DO—EXTERNAL APPLICATIONS

- Avoid washing with regular soaps and shampoos, or using baby oils. Bathe affected parts often with plain water. Afterward rub with a slice of cucumber. Apply lanolin-based ointment fortified with Vitamin A and E oils or pure Aloe Vera gel.
- Mix one part Sage oil with ten parts Olive oil and apply locally.
- Dusting with Whey powder can be soothing.
- Seawater can be beneficial, especially combined with careful exposure to the sun.
- For a hot inflamed type of eczema, add ¼ cup baking soda to bath 2–3 times weekly and soak in it for 15 minutes.
- For a dry, itchy type of eczema, add ¼ cup powdered Ginger to bath 2–3 times weekly and soak in it for 15 minutes.

HERBS

These may cause an initial worsening of the condition due to increased elimination of toxins. Do not introduce any new creams at the same time as it may interfere with the cleansing process.

Blood purifiers: Burdock, Dandelion, Yellow Dock, Elecampane, Echinacea, and/or Sassafras
Bowel cleaners: Black Walnut or Rosemary

HOMEOPATHIC

Arsen Alb 30c: Chronic dry eczema with great burning and itching, thickened skin.
Graphites 30c: Raw behind ears, hands, elbow and knee flexures; cracks in nipples, toes, mouth, or anus. Sticky, scabby eruptions oozing a gluey, honeylike fluid.
Nat Mur 30c: Raw, red, and inflamed. Worse from eating salt or at the seashore.

Psorinum 30c: Intolerable itching all night, inherited tendency. Erupts on bends of joints with itching. Worse from warmth of bed. Very greasy, dirty-looking skin.

Rhus Tox 30c: Acute intense itching and tingling; red, swollen, circular shaped, and scaly; better from warm applications.

Sulphur 30c: Dry and scaly; itching and burning; worse from scratching and washing, every injury becomes infected. Skin troubles alternate with intestinal problems.

There may be an initial worsening of symptoms due to increased elimination of toxins. Discontinue remedy immediately if this occurs and wait for things to settle down.

CELL SALTS

Kali Mur: Skin has white, dry scales.

Kali Phos: Good for nervous children; skin is raw and sore.

Kali Sulph: Discharge is yellow looking.

Nat Mur: Watery eruptions worse in folds such as elbows and knees; skin is itchy, dry, and cracked.

Emergency Techniques

When a person is partially or completely unconscious:

- Do not give anything to drink. (Homeopathic remedies can be given as they are absorbed through the mucous membranes of the mouth.)
- Do not leave unattended.
- Do not move unless this is vital to life.
- Send someone to contact medical help immediately. Proceed with Ten Steps for Casualty Care below.

For emergency use of homeopathy, see page 114.

TEN STEPS FOR CASUALTY CARE

1. Guard against further danger

    Building collapse: Beware of other dangers: live wires, gas leak, etc.

    Electric shock: Switch off power or move child from power source using a wooden-handled broom. Beware of any water.

    Gas: Don't breathe in fumes yourself. Open doors and drag child to safety if possible.

    Machinery: Stop the machine.

    Road accidents: Protect yourself and others from oncoming cars. Is damaged car safe from fire or falling?

    Under heavy objects: Don't lift object unless you are sure you are able to lift it clear of child.

2. Airways

    Is the child breathing? If not, she will die unless breathing is restored:

    - Undo tight clothing from neck, chest, and waist.
    - Clear obstruction from the mouth, such as vomit, loose teeth. (Turn head to one side and scoop out debris, using two fingers.)
    - Check also that tongue does not block the airways. (For adults, do *not* remove false teeth.)
    - Tilt head by placing one hand under the neck and the other across the forehead. Push neck up gently and tilt head back so chin juts up.
    - Give four quick breaths into the child's mouth and nose to inflate their lungs. Remember: Your lungs are larger than a child's, so adjust your breath accordingly.

3. Breathing

    If breathing does not return automatically after above procedure, begin Artificial Respiration.

    Keeping child's head tilted with chin up:

- Open your mouth and take a breath.
- Seal your mouth around the child's mouth and nose; for larger child, pinch nose and puff gently into mouth.
- Puff gently into child's lungs until chest rises.
- Remove your mouth and watch the child's chest fall. Turn your head slightly so as to avoid his/her expelled air—you will quickly tire if you don't get fresh air yourself; also, if the child has inhaled a toxic gas it is well to avoid breathing in her expelled air.
- Repeat until normal breathing returns.

4. Circulation

   Is the child's heart beating? Place two fingers in the groove of the neck alongside the Adam's apple or place your ear on the child's breastbone and listen for heartbeat. If you are sure there is no pulse, proceed with CPR (Cardio-Pulmonary Resuscitation, or Cardiac Massage). CPR should be done by a person who has been trained in the technique. If you have not been trained and there is no one with you who has been trained, proceed *carefully* with the following instructions:

   (1) Position yourself alongside child, who should be on her back on a firm surface.

   (2) Perform massage:

   Under one year: Place two fingers on lower breastbone (bone down the middle of the chest where the ribs meet) and push this down ($\frac{1}{2}$ inch), then release. Continue regularly at about 100 depressions per minute (1-and-2-and 3-and-4-and-etc.).

   Children 1–10 years: Place heel of one hand on center of lower half of breastbone and push this down (1 inch), then release. Repeat regularly at about 80–90 depressions per minute (1-rabbit-2-rabbit-3-rabbit-4-rabbit).

   Children over 10 and Adults: Position your body above and slightly over the child. Place heel of one hand on center of lower half of breastbone. Place heel of other hand on top and interlock fingers of two hands together. Keeping arms straight and fingers clear of chest, press firmly straight down toward the floor, depressing bone (1½–2 inches). Release, then repeat regularly at about 60 depressions per minute (1-crocodile-2-crocodile-3-crocodile-4-crocodile-5-crocodile).

If one rescuer: Give fifteen compressions of the heart, then two rescue breaths. Repeat this cycle, checking pulse every fourth cycle.

If two rescuers: Give five compressions of the heart, then one rescue breath. Repeat this cycle, checking pulse after every twelve cycles.

Continue until automatic breathing starts again, and pulse returns. As soon as heartbeat returns, stop compression. When resuscitation is successful, the child's face color will improve, becoming more pink and less blue. Continue to check both breathing and pulse regularly until help arrives.

Recovery Position: If there are no other signs of injury, place child in Recovery Position. This position may not be ideal if you suspect a spinal injury, however it must be used immediately if breathing becomes difficult or if child must be left unattended.

5. Bleeding
   Deal first with wounds that are:

- Producing a lot of blood.
- Spurting bright red (arterial) blood.
- To the chest, where air is being sucked in and out of the wound during breathing. Seal the "hole" quickly as otherwise child will suffocate. Raise head and shoulders slightly.

(1) Your first objective is to stop the bleeding. Elevate the part (if possible) unless fracture is suspected. Apply *direct pressure* over and around the wound using bandages or pads to constrict the blood vessels in the area. Maintain pressure for 5–15 minutes. If

bleeding cannot be controlled by direct pressure, then apply *indirect pressure* to one of the larger arteries:

(a) Brachial artery on the inside of the upper arm: Press up and in under the arm pushing the artery against the bone. Use this method for excessive bleeding on the arm but do not apply pressure for more than 15 minutes.

(b) Femoral artery on the inside of the upper leg. Press in and upward where the thigh meets the groin with your fist or the heel of your hand against the rim of the pelvis. Use this method for excessive bleeding anywhere on the leg. Do not maintain pressure for more than 15 minutes.

SEEK MEDICAL HELP IMMEDIATELY.

(2) Cover wound with clean light dressing soaked in Hypercal solution (10 drops to half-glass water). Follow with a pad of cotton or clean linen.

(3) Bandage firmly until further treatment (see Wounds). Elevate the part.

If sharp object or bone is protruding from wound: Do not remove object or push back bone. Mold pads of clean material around the wound to a height that will prevent pressure on object or bone. Bandage diagonally between the wound and the heart to slow bleeding. *Don't press on object or bone.*

Abdominal wounds: These may not bleed profusely but there may be internal damage. *Do not push back any internal organs that are protruding*—protect them with a clean light covering and SEEK MEDICAL HELP IMMEDIATELY. DO NOT GIVE ANYTHING TO DRINK. (Homeopathic remedies can be given as they are absorbed through mucous membranes of the mouth).

6. Medical Help

Contact medical help at this stage if not already called. Dial emergency phone number and ask for an ambulance.

7. Fractures

Immobilize fractures or broken bones (see Fractures, page 126).

8. Shock

Treat child for shock (see Shock, page 195).

9. Position

Do not move a child who has already been placed in the Recovery Position. In less serious cases, place child in most comfortable position consistent with the requirements of treatment.

10. Check

Continue to check breathing, heart, and injuries until help arrives.

UNCONSCIOUSNESS

Attempt to work out the cause of the child's unconsciousness to report to medical help. The most common causes are poison; car accident; head injury; shock; stroke; epilepsy; convulsions; diabetes (refer to appropriate headings, if necessary).

LEVELS OF RESPONSIVENESS

Unconsciousness is caused by some interference with the normal functions of the nervous system and circulation. It may develop slowly through progressive levels of unconsciousness:

Drowsiness: Easily roused but lapses back into unconsciousness, answers questions normally.

Stupor: Can be roused but with difficulty, cannot answer questions normally but does feel physical stimuli.

Coma: Cannot be roused.

Every 10 minutes you should recheck the child's response level, e.g.,

- to noise (by speaking loudly).
- to touch (by gently shaking).
- to pain (by pinching skin).

- to reflex (by touching eyelashes) and record your findings.

SEEK MEDICAL AID if you have not already done so.

Emergency Use of Homeopathy

For emergency first-aid techniques (artificial respiration and CPR), see pages 109 and 110.
IF THE CONDITION IS SERIOUS, CALL AN AMBULANCE.

DESCRIPTION

Homeopathy offers quiet, effective help while medical aid is on its way. Its remedies are absorbed through the mucous membranes of the mouth and so are safe to give to an unconscious person.

WHAT TO DO

Arnica 30c or 200c: The first remedy to use, as it helps the body react to trauma in the best possible way. Place 4 drops on tongue or crush a tablet (between spoons if available), mix with a little water, then place a few drops inside lips.

Arnica 30c can be repeated as often as every few minutes if the situation is critical, doubling the time between doses as the condition improves. For a less critical condition, remedy can be repeated at 15–minute intervals, then double the time between doses as condition improves.

SPECIFIC SITUATIONS

- See under individual headings:

Bloody nose, page 171   Head injuries, page 134

Burns, page 66

Choking, page 72

Convulsions (fits), page 124

Eye injuries, page 117

Fractures, page 126

Hemorrhage (bleeding), page 111

Heat exhaustion, page 135

Heat stroke, page 135

Poisoning, page 177

Shock, page 195

- Other emergencies:

Asphyxia (lack of oxygen, irregular breathing, blue/purplish skin color): Clear airway, prop open jaws with cork, do CPR (cardiac massage—see page 110) if necessary.

Antim Tart 30c: Pale face, cold and sweaty, rattling breathing, can't get breath.

Apis 30c: If breathing difficulty is caused by sudden severe swelling of tongue or throat.

Carbo Veg 30c: Puffy blue face with cold sweat, collapse, and air hunger.

Collapse (fainting; gray ashen color; cold clammy skin, shallow breathing, falling temperature, rising pulse, restless): Loosen tight clothing, open windows, give no drink if unconscious.

Aconite 30c: Collapse with great anxiety and fear.

Arnica 30c: When collapse is caused by injury or hemorrhage.

Carbo Veg 30c: Cold breath, great gasping for air; desire to be fanned yet cold.

Veratrum Alb 30c: Skin is very cold. Cold sweat on forehead.

Frostbite (excessive chilling of extremities, causing initial numbness and maybe permanent tissue damage): Do not rub. Keep affected part warm next to your skin.

Apis 30c: If stinging burning and swelling occur.

Lachesis 30c: Extremities lose sensation and become discolored.

Spinal injuries

Hypericum 30c: To prevent potential back problems or concussion after fall or crushing injury to spine.

Stroke (a hemorrhage of the brain that might be slight or severe).

Aconite 30c: For confusion, shock, numbness. Follow with Arnica 30C at regular intervals. Continue with Arnica three times daily for many weeks, if severe.

Sunburn (red tender skin, may be followed by blistering; from overexposure to the sun).

Cantharis 30c: For intense burning at first stage before blisters have formed.
Urtica Urens 30c: For burns accompanied by intense stinging. For Sunstroke, see page 135.

SURGICAL OPERATIONS

Arnica 30c: Three doses before and three doses after operation. Repeat if required. Drops are best.
Aconite 30c: If prospect of operation is causing excessive fear.
Hypericum 30c: For sharp shooting pains.
Phosphorus 30c: For vomiting after operation (caused by anesthetic).
Staphysagria 30c: For severe pain after operation (especially for circumcision, dental operations).

Eyes

1 Object in Eye
2 Blow to Eye
3 Sty

4 Blocked Tear Duct

5 Eyestrain and Poor Vision

6 Squint

7 Danger Signs with Eyes

1 Object in Eye

- If object is embedded in the eyeball, do *not* attempt to remove. Give Aconite 30c for shock and irritation and SEEK MEDICAL ADVICE.
- If object is freely moving in the eye, hold eyelids open, and using a cotton swab or corner of a clean handkerchief, gently wipe object from eye.
- If child will not allow this, place one drop of Castor oil in eye to move object. After it is removed, apply firm pressure over closed eye using a soft pad such as a folded clean handkerchief.
- If eye is painful and child will not allow you to touch it, it is best to get your doctor or local hospital to use pain-relieving eye drops and remove it for you.
- For bleeding, bathe with Hypercal solution (made with five drops to half a glass of water, or one drop to an eye bath of water).
- If eye remains bloodshot or sore over the next few days, take Ruta Grav 30c three times during the day.

2 Blow to Eye

All blows to the eye are potentially serious.
- If very severe, *do not examine* as this may aggravate the situation. Rest in lying down position. Apply cold compress immediately. Make compress (see page 7) using Comfrey or Eyebright; or Arnica tincture (diluted five drops to half-cup of water).
- Keep eye covered with dressing but do not apply pressure.
- SEEK MEDICAL ADVICE if blow is severe. The eye can fill with blood. This can lead to glaucoma, so watch for bleeding

behind the cornea.

- Take Arnica 30c internally for a few days to reduce the blackening and swelling.

3 Sty

An infection at the base of hairs that form eyelashes. Starts as redness and tender swelling, then pus forms and can discharge. Conjunctivitis can develop.

WHAT TO DO

At first feeling of tenderness or redness, gently pull at eyelashes. This can remove the loose hair and irritation sometimes subsides. Make a solution with 10 drops of Hypercal or Euphrasia tincture in half a glass of water (or one drop to eye bath) and wash eye and eyelid at least three times daily.

HERBS

Eye can be bathed with Chamomile tea.

Eyebright, Golden Seat, and Bayberry can be taken together as a tea 3–4 times daily. These herbs are all beneficial for the eyes.

HOMEOPATHIC

Aconite 30c: Inflamed from cold and feels like sand is in the eye. Worse from cold, dry winds. Sensitive to light.

Apis 30c: To help prevent recurrence.

Graphites 30c: Red, swollen lids, worse from light.

Hepar Sulph 30c: For chronic sty problems. Worse from cold air and cold applications.

Pulsatilla 30c: For sties on the lower lid. Thick yellow bland discharge.

Silica 30c: Swollen tear ducts, worse from sunlight. Pustular condition about eyes.

Sulphur 30c: Burning ulceration of lids.

Silica.

4 Blocked Tear Duct

There are more tears in one eye and there may be yellow discharge.

WHAT TO DO

Gently massage down cheek from inner lower edge of eye below tear duct. Repeat twice daily.

HOMEOPATHIC

Calc Carb 30c: Eye waters more in open air and early morning.
Nat Mur 30c: If discharge is more yellow and irritating.

CELL SALTS

Nat Mur.

5 Eyestrain and Poor Vision

Some children complain of tired eyes after school or television. Some children with poor vision never complain, so be sure your child's vision is checked at school and learn to make your own observations. Watch for:

- Difficulty reading the blackboard.
- Holding books very close to the eyes.
- Sitting very close to the television.
- Developing headaches or pain around eyes.

WHAT TO DO

Eye exercises and Touch for Health techniques can be useful. See an instructor and check with an opthalmologist.

HERBS

To relieve eyestrain: Eyebright, Golden Seal, and Bayberry. (A weaker tea made from these can also be used as an eyewash.)

To strengthen: Jaborandi, Parsley, or Chaparral. Vitamin A has a specific affinity for the eyes.

HOMEOPATHIC

Causticum 30c: Sparks and dark spots, film before eyes, feeling of pressure in eyeballs. Muscular weakness, double vision.

China 30c: Black specks, bright dazzling before eyes, feeling of pressure in eyeballs.

Gelsemium 30c: Heavy or stiff eyelids. Maybe double vision from paralysis of eyelids.

Nat Mur 30c: Letters run together; zigzag shapes; pain on looking down. Much watering and scalding.

Phosphorus 30c: Letters look red, spots before eyes. Cloudiness, or green halo about objects.

Ruta Grav 30c: Red, hot, painful eyes from sewing or reading. Blurred vision. Eyestrain is followed by headache.

CELL SALTS

Calc Fluor: Blurred vision from eyestrain.
Ferr Phos: Pain from overstraining eyes.
Kali Phos: Weak eyesight from ill health.

6 Squint

The eyes look in different directions at the same time.

HOMEOPATHIC

Belladonna 30c: Squint sometimes with staring, fiery eyes in an excitable child.

Cicuta 30c: Spasmodic squint, pupils can move behind upper lids when head bends back.

7 Danger Signs with Eyes

SEEK PROFESSIONAL ADVICE FOR:

- Any wound, cut, or foreign body that enters eyeball.
- A painful, grayish spot on cornea with redness around cornea.
- Pain inside eye—iritis or glaucoma.
- Difference in pupil size, especially with pain or headache.
- Vision changing or fading.
- Any inflammation or infection that fails to respond to treatment (whether medical or natural).
- If condition fails to respond to above procedures.

Fever

When the body is upset by some invasion, whether the common cold virus or something more serious, the temperature will rise.

All healing processes speed up during a fever—the heart carrying blood, the respiration increasing oxygen uptake. Fever is not an enemy to be suppressed, but a signal that the body is working to ward off an invasion. With children under five years, a rise in temperature can produce a "fever fit" (see Fits), so it is important to keep the temperature below danger level while not suppressing it entirely.

Mild Fever: 99.5–101°F.
Moderate Fever: 101–103°F.
High: 103° F This temperature should be lowered quickly.
Extremely High: over 104°F This temperature must be cooled
    at once, to avoid convulsions.

WHAT TO DO

- Cool: Strip child to underclothes; if still hot to touch, sponge gently with tepid water or put in a tepid bath. Extreme cooling by cold baths causes the body to react against being chilled, i.e., triggers the heating mechanisms. However, with a temperature of 104°F or more, iced water is appropriate.

- Give child frequent, small drinks of water and herbal teas (see below).
- Find the cause of the fever and take steps to correct this.

HERBS

Herbs are best prepared hot and given frequently for fevers.
Laxative herbs to help eliminate toxic matter through the bowel: Senna, Thyme or Licorice. Use these only if the child is constipated.

To help bring down fever: Yarrow, Lemon Balm, Catnip, and/or Ginger
To the bath: Add 1–2 Tbs. Ginger powder or Epsom salts; or 2–3 drops of oils of Peppermint, Sage, and/or Thyme.

HOMEOPATHIC

Homeopathic remedies provide a good first action that may often allay a more serious illness.

Aconite 30c: Sudden onset in a normally healthy child. Intensely nervous, restless, anxious. Skin is dry and hot with full, bounding pulse. Red cheeks; chilly on slightest movement. Great thirst.
Antim Tart 30c: Shivering with fever, pale face, thirst for little sips often. Chilly with short burst of heat.
Arsen Alb 30c: Patient is fearful and restless, burning pains relieved by warmth. Very thirsty for frequent sips, rapid prostration, and increasing weakness.
Belladonna 30c: Sudden, violent onset. Flushed face, high temperature, pulse strong and rapid. Little or no thirst, may be delirious. Dry, burning hot skin, sparkling eyes.
Bryonia 30c: Fever with intense headache; prefers to lie still. Worse from least movement, even moving eyes. Very thirsty for large drinks of water. Pale and quiet. White coating down middle of tongue.
China 30c: May help the child who develops a fever easily and often.

Gelsemium 30c: Chilly, aches all over. Dizzy; does not want to move, dull headache, droopy eyes, heavy limbs, no thirst.

Mercurius 30c: Alternatively hot and cold. Profuse perspiration with no relief. Worse at night.

Rhus Tox 30c: Great weakness and prostration but extremely restless. Mental confusion, thickly coated tongue, but red at tip, great thirst.

CELL SALTS

Ferr Phos: First remedy for high temperature. Gradual onset. Red cheeks and throbbing head. Fast pulse. Better from cold applications to head.

Kali Phos: For those with a nervous temperature, this seems more effective than Ferr Phos.

SEEK MEDICAL ADVICE

If temperature remains above 103°F despite procedure. See also Fits, page 124.

First Aid

See **Emergency, p. 108.**

Fits

Fits or convulsions occur when the brain sends out jumbled messages to the muscles, making them move in uncontrolled ways. Fits usually last only a few minutes and are not uncommon between six months and three years, but are rare after five years. They are usually accompanied by a fever.

If children have had one fever fit, they are more susceptible to such fits. (If your child is having fits frequently without any sign of fever, then epilepsy is a possibility—seek medical, homeopathic, or naturopathic advice.)

Convulsions can occur during meningitis (see Meningitis).

DESCRIPTION

Child can sometimes be only slightly unwell and temperature rises very quickly. During the fit, the child goes stiff, eyes roll back, breathing is labored, body twitches and shakes, child may turn blue around lips or bite tongue.

Child becomes unconscious, may vomit or soil himself; body relaxes and as he regains consciousness, he is confused. After a sleep he wakens fully recovered.

WHAT TO DO

- Keep child cool (with fever fits this is most important—see Fever).
- Place gently on side (in Recovery or coma position—see Emergency) to prevent choking.
- Remove anything from in front of child's mouth.
- Ensure he cannot hurt himself.
- Remove tight clothing from neck.
- After fit has finished, reassure and comfort child.

DURING FIT

HERBS

Place on tongue: 1–2 drops of Chamomile, Valerian, Lavender, or Skullcap tincture. Repeat every few minutes.

HOMEOPATHIC

Aconite 30c: If convulsions are caused by a fright. Rigid and stiff with bright red face, foaming at mouth, crying out in sleep.
Belladonna 30c: Violent onset with large, glazed pupils.

Cuprum 30c: Violent convulsions with contraction of jaws; may begin in fingers or toes. Blue face and mouth. Gurgling in throat.

Ignatia 30c: For child who becomes hysterical due to grief, worry, jealousy, or after punishment. Twitching muscles.

Zincum 30c: Convulsion following infection or fever.

CELL SALTS

Place on tongue one crushed Mag Phos tablet; follow in a few minutes with Calc Phos. Continue to alternate during convulsion and follow with 2–3 doses afterward as well.

LONG-TERM APPROACH

If your child has had any fits, give daily drinks of Skullcap, Valerian, and/or Passionflower to calm the nervous system. Continue thirty days.

SEEK MEDICAL ADVICE:

- If it is child's first fever fit.
- If child comes out of one fit and goes straight into another, despite above procedure.
- If child continues to have fits despite above procedure.

Fractures

After a child has had a fall, check for the following:

- Painful swelling in any area other than bruised part.
- One point of extreme tenderness over a bone.
- A change in body shape on one side but not the other.

- Child is unable to use a limb.
- If pulse cannot be felt beyond an injury.

WHAT TO DO

1. If child has severe bleeding or shows signs of shock always deal with these first (see Wounds or Emergency).
2. SEEK MEDICAL HELP IMMEDIATELY.
3. Immobilize injured part by strapping firmly with strips of cloth or diapers and supporting limb wherever possible with splint, e.g., rolled- up newspaper), or strap to uninjured part of body.
4. Support in an elevated position when possible.
5. Never put an exposed broken bone (compound fracture) back into the wound—expert aid is required to thoroughly clean the area.

HERBS

Taken internally to help broken bones heal

To calm nerves and ease pain: Chamomile or Valerian
To ensure adequate Calcium and Magnesium during healing: Basil and Parsley
To help heal: Comfrey

Externally

Apply Comfrey ointment to unbroken skin to help swelling, deformity, and unnatural mobility.

HOMEOPATHIC

Arnica 30c: 3–4 times daily for first three days.
Symphytum 6x: Take twice daily for the first three weeks to help unite fracture.
Bryonia 30c: If swelling is great.
Hypericum 30c: For pain caused by damage to nerves.

Ruta Grav 30c: May be taken for pain in injured bones.

CELL SALTS

Calc Phos: To help unite fracture.
Alternate with Ferr Phos when there is redness and/or swelling around injury.

SEEK IMMEDIATE MEDICAL HELP for fracture to skull, face, or jaw. If there is bloody or straw-colored discharge from ear, place pad over ear and secure lightly; watch breathing; check airways for tongue, swollen tissue, or other blockages; give Artificial Respiration (see Emergency p.108), if necessary.

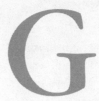

Glands

Lymph glands are special organs of varying sizes, situated in many parts of the body, for the purpose of obstructing foreign particles, disease germs, and chemical poisons from entering or remaining in the bloodstream.

Any harmful materials trapped in the glands produce an enlargement of the gland, which can easily be seen and felt if the affected gland is close to the body surface. These swellings may be painful and tender if they are caused by inflammation or if they come on rapidly. If the enlargement is slow, the swellings are usually without pain.

DESCRIPTION

Many glands swollen and inflamed either together or appearing in succession may indicate acute infectious disease such as scarlet fever, glandular fever, smallpox, typhoid, Hodgkin's disease, severe systemic infection, German measles, leukemia, or generalized skin infections.

Swollen tender glands in the neck or under the jaws may indicate an infected or congested throat, mouth or ear, bad cold in the nose, or mumps. Swollen glands in the armpits may indicate infection or congestion in the arm, hand, or breast area.

Swollen glands in the groin may indicate infection or congestion on feet, legs, genital organs, anus, or buttocks.

Swollen glands on back of neck may indicate infection or congestion on the scalp.

WHAT TO DO

Seek advice when many glands are swollen. At the same time, any natural approach will be of benefit to help rid the body of the harmful materials.

NOTE: The importance of lymph glands should not be overlooked when removal of tonsils and adenoids is being considered. If seriously infected, or enlarged enough to interfere with breathing or swallowing, they may need surgical removal. Otherwise, they should be left in their proper places to perform their normal function of catching and sifting out harmful matter.

HERBS

To fight off an infection and help eliminate poisons, the body benefits from herbs rich in Vitamins A, B, C, and E, which are usually found lacking in such circumstances. Combine any of the following herbs and drink small amounts often, throughout the day: Rosemary, Comfrey, Elder, Mullein, Honeysuckle, Golden Seal, Echinacea, and Poke Root.

HOMEOPATHIC

There are many remedies for swollen glands. Included here are the most common, as recommended in our health kit (page 6). See a homeopath for further advice, if required.

Baryta Carb 30c: For chronic swelling of glands of neck, throat, abdomen, underarms, around ears.

Belladonna 30c: For acute swellings that are red, painful, and sudden.

Calc Carb 30c: For swollen glands accompanied by bad breath and putrid body odor in a child who perspires and tends to put on weight easily. Worse from cold water or wet weather.

Carbo An 30c: Hard, stony glands of neck, underarms, groin, breast area accompanied by cutting, burning pains.

Silica 30c: For inflamed, swollen glands that develop slowly and become septic.

CELL SALTS

Ferr Phos: For the fever and pain accompanying acute inflammations and ulcerated glands.

Calc Fluor: For stony, hard swellings.

Kali Mur: For soft, inflamed swellings of neck, adenoids, throat, and salivary glands.

Silica: For swollen, pus-filled sebaceous glands. (These are the oil-secreting glands of the skin that, when infected, cause blackheads, pimples, pustules, etc.)

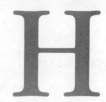

Headache

Headache can be caused by any of the following: spinal problems, visual strain, blood sugar problems, stress, muscular tension, digestive disturbances, allergies, sinusitis, cranial faults, dehydration, or infection, e.g., influenza, measles.

A *migraine* is a severe headache often occurring at regular intervals, usually one-sided and accompanied by nausea, vomiting, and may be preceded or accompanied by visual disturbances.

WHAT TO DO—INTERNAL APPLICATIONS

The information here applies to both headaches and migraines. If you suspect a spinal or neck problem, check with a qualified osteopath or chiropractor.

Dietary changes may be necessary, but such changes vary from person to person. See Allergy, or seek advice from a naturopath, homeopath, or Touch for Health instructor. Simple avoidance of fried foods, sugar products, and dairy products may help—and remember to drink small amounts of water often.

HERBS

Choose at least one from each of the following categories and make a tea to be sipped often during headache.

For nerves: Valerian, Skullcap, Passionflower, or Thyme.

To regulate blood sugar and liver action: Meadowsweet, Dandelion, Mandrake, and/or Golden Seal.

To strengthen and harmonize the digestive system: Fennel, Sage, Rosemary, Thyme, Lavender, and/or Peppermint.

WHAT TO DO—EXTERNAL APPLICATIONS

To soothe: A few drops of oil of Rose or Lemongrass in the bath.

HOMEOPATHIC

Argentum Nit 30c: Head feels extremely large; dizziness, better for pressure to head.

Belladonna 30c: Hot head; throbbing flushed face and cold feet; right front of head worse for lying down, uncovering, light, noise, jar; better for holding head still or bending head backwards.

Bryonia 30c: Bursting, splitting frontal ache; extends backward down neck and shoulders. Worse for moving eyes, and in the morning.

China 30c: Head feels as if brain is bouncing within skull. Better from bending double.

Gelsemium 30c: Heavy eyelids, dull heavy ache with dizziness; tight band feeling around head, worse from emotion or bad news.

Nat Mur 30c: Blinding headache with pale face and nausea, preceded by numbness and tingling in lips, tongue and nose. Worse from eyestrain, better after sleep. Sensation as if little hammers were beating in head.

Nux Vomica 30c: Headache with retching, vomiting, and often constipation, worse in morning; either at back of head or over one eye.

CELL SALTS

Ferr Phos: Headache with bloodshot eyes; often accompanies a cold.

Kali Phos: Headache with bad breath, brown-coated tongue, worse from noise and lack of sleep; child may be nervous, excitable type.

Mag Phos: Headache with eye troubles; sparks before eyes; shooting pains into head.

Nat Mur: Dull, heavy head with watering eyes and constipation.

SEEK MEDICAL, HOMEOPATHIC, OR NATUROPATHIC ADVICE if headaches are severe, or recur frequently.

See also: **Allergy, Eyestrain, Digestive Problems, Influenza, Meningitis, Hepatitis, Measles, Stomach.**

Head Injury

Any blow to the head may cause concussion (temporary disturbance of brain function), so watch carefully for symptoms as outlined below. For *wounds* to the head, see Wounds, page 228.

WHAT TO DO

HOMEOPATHIC

After any blow to the head, give Nat Sulph 30c, alternating at 15–minute intervals with Arnica 200c for the first hour. (During an acute condition, the body makes quicker use of the remedies, therefore the time between them can be considerably less than usual.) Continue with Arnica 30c three times daily for a few days.

Check the symptoms below for the next twenty-four hours; rouse the child several times during the first night if it was a heavy blow, to ensure the child is not unconscious. If necessary, follow up with:

Aconite 30c: If the child shows fear and shock.

Nat Sulph 200c: For lingering aftereffects of a head injury (for 200c potency, see page 13).

CELL SALTS

Ferr Phos and Kali Phos mixed together can be given in the same day, four times in twenty-four hours.

Nat Sulph: Head injury with dizziness. Give every fifteen minutes.

SEEK MEDICAL ADVICE

- If there is any unconsciousness, no matter how brief.
- If despite above procedure there is any deterioration at all.
- If child shows signs of *concussion*. These are:

  - Pupils unequal
  - Starts to become sleepy or woozy
  - Hard to rouse from sleep
  - Pulse rate goes up
  - Vision is disturbed
  - Difficulty moving any limb
  - Signs of a headache
  - If a blow is followed by bloody or straw-colored discharge from ear (possible skull fracture)

Heat Exhaustion/Heatstroke

A profound failure of the circulation to regulate the temperature level. May be brought on by high atmospheric temperatures; high humidity with low air current; excessive sweating through exercise; or inability to sweat, poor ventilation, overcrowding, being overdressed (babies or toddlers), high fever (e.g., malaria). Sunstroke can mark the beginning of heatstroke.

DESCRIPTION—HEAT EXHAUSTION

Weakness, faintness, profuse sweating but stable temperature; large pupils; pale, cool skin; muscle cramps. Fast shallow breathing; rapid, weak pulse.

WHAT TO DO

Place child at rest in a cool place; elevate legs.

Due to loss of salt and minerals, give electrolyte solution (or make up ½ tsp. salt, 8 tsp. sugar/honey in 2.1 cups boiled water). Take as frequent small drinks.

Avoid reexposure to heat. Watch for shock reaction.

DESCRIPTION—HEATSTROKE

Vomiting, headache, nausea; red, hot, and dry skin—not even armpits are moist; increase in temperature pulse; drowsiness; maybe diarrhea. In serious cases there may be delirium and eventually unconsciousness. Heatstroke can be very dangerous.

WHAT TO DO

- *This is an emergency.* SEEK MEDICAL AID.
- Cool the body as rapidly as possible with tepid sponging or lukewarm bath. Alternatively, wrap body in cold wet sheet and keep wet with ice or sprayed water. Fan continually, keep child upright.
- If temperature is over 104°F, use cold water.
- If temperature is over 107.6°F, use iced water if possible. Give plenty of small drinks of water or unsweetened juice.
- Place at rest in a cool place.
- Ensure child does not become overheated during the next few weeks.

FOR BOTH HEAT EXHAUSTION AND HEATSTROKE

HERBS

To help stabilize the temperature levels and provide adequate Vitamins C and E: Lavender, Rosemary, Skullcap, and Lemon Balm can be sipped often. These can be taken together or separately.

HOMEOPATHIC

Belladonna 30c: Bounding pulse, delirium, burning red hot and dry skin. Pupils are dilated and fixed.

Bryonia 30c: Splitting headache, worse from sitting up and moving about which makes child nauseated.

China 30c: Great exhaustion brought on by excessive sweating; hot face with cold hands.

Cuprum Met 30c: When accompanied by convulsions and severe cramps.

Gelsemium 30c: Worse from exposure to sun; recurrent fever and weakness; tired eyes and limbs, depression.

Glonoine 30c: Surging of blood to head and neck; sees sparks; throbbing headache worse from heat, hot flushed face and sweaty skin.

Mezereum 30c: Give night and morning before exposure, for those who are greatly affected by the heat.

Hepatitis

An inflammation of the liver that can be caused by a variety of agents such as infections, toxic drugs, and poisons.

A notifiable disease—must be reported to a medical doctor or local health department.

Hepatitis A is infectious, occurring sporadically or in epidemics; transmitted orally by hand or by flies contaminated by the bowel movements of a person with hepatitis.

Hepatitis B is serum hepatitis transmitted via blood products.

DESCRIPTION—HEPATITIS A

Quick onset; gastrointestinal disturbance, fever, lack of appetite, aching in back and limbs, vomiting, diarrhea, itchy skin, weight loss. Jaundice (yellowing of skin and eyes) appears as other symptoms improve. Depression and tiredness can persist for some months. If symptoms persist for six months or more after an acute attack, this is known as chronic hepatitis.

Incubation period: 30–40 days.
Isolation period: Until fever subsides.
Recovery rate: 3–16 weeks.

DESCRIPTION—HEPATITIS B

Sudden onset; headache, fever, chills, general weakness, nausea, vomiting, abdominal pains, jaundice. Depression and tiredness can persist for some months. If symptoms persist for six months or more after an acute attack, this is known as chronic hepatitis.

Incubation period: 41–108 days.

DESCRIPTION—HEPATITIS C

Transmitted by blood contact, constant lower resistance to infection, has higher incidence of liver damage in the long term.

WHAT TO DO

The same approach applies to all forms of hepatitis.
- Bed rest is essential for at least two weeks.
- Avoid physical exertion, unnecessary travel, and strong medication wherever possible.

- Food is best kept to a bare minimum. Use fresh fruits and vegetables if child is hungry.
- Avoid fried foods, fatty foods, egg yolks, excess protein, and alcohol.
- Beetroot, carrot and dandelion juices are especially beneficial. Freshly squeezed citrus juice mixed with water (1:1) should be sipped daily.

HERBS

As antiseptic: Golden Seal or Thyme
For diarrhea: Meadowsweat, Raspberry
For depression: Gotu Kola, St. Johns Wort
For extra nourishment: Lemon and Rosemary
To restore energy: Gentian
To strengthen the liver: Barberry, Mandrake, and/or Yarrow, Milk Thistle (helps build new cells), Licorice, Fennel, Dandelion, Burdock

HOMEOPATHIC

It is better to use the tablets (lactose based) than the drops (alcohol based), which might add extra strain to the liver.
After suspected contact, see Resistance and Immunity, page 19.

Bryonia 30c: Child is irritable, nauseous and dizzy. Liver is swollen with stitching pain in upper right side of abdomen and under right shoulder blade: bitter taste in mouth. Child is worse from motion, better lying on right side.
Chelidonium 30c: Sore stitching pain in liver; pain under liver and lower angle of right shoulder blade; fever, chills, and diarrhea.
China 30c: Shooting, pressing pain in liver; liver feels swollen and hard; tongue has thick, yellow coating with bitter taste.
Hepar Sulph 30c: Irritable; heaviness and pressure after slight meal, stitching in liver worse from walking, laughing, breathing, pressure.

Mercurius 30c: Liver swollen and sore to touch; stabbing pain, cannot lie on right side; teeth imprints on yellow tongue; foul breath.

Nat Sulph 30c: Bursting feeling in head with burning in stomach; vomiting of bile; aching, cutting pain in liver, yellow complexion and eyes, cannot bear anything tight around waist; worse lying on left side.

Hepatitis A or Hepatitis B 200c Nosode: Can be given but this is best after dietary changes have been made and liver-strengthening herbs have been taken for several months.

CELL SALTS

Kali Mur: Jaundice with constipation, swollen liver, white-coated tongue, lack of appetite, light-colored stools and headache.

Nat Sulph: Liver is sore, congested; child is yellow, vomits bile, and has a greenish coating on tongue.

LONG-TERM APPROACH

If child continues to remain tired and depressed after hepatitis, continue with above herbs and dietary recommendations daily.

Calc Phos 6x can be very helpful if child develops symptoms of twitching, jerking, itching, and weakness. Give twice daily for several weeks.

TO BUILD RESISTANCE

To help strengthen the immune system and restore to full health after disease or vaccination, see page 19.

Hernia

A protrusion of any part of the internal organs through the structures enclosing them.

Hiatus Hernia: Stomach protrudes through diaphragm.

Inguinal Hernia: Intestine protrudes through the inguinal canal (i.e., muscles in groin).

Strangulated Hernia: The protruding part becomes pinched and passage of material through intestine is stopped.

Umbilical Hernia: Intestinal loop protrudes through the umbilicus (belly button).

DESCRIPTION

A lump or swelling in any part of the aforementioned areas, causing discomfort made worse by coughing or after eating. There is pain, heartburn, vomiting, or acid regurgitation. Usually a person with a hernia has had a weak spot in the muscle that gradually worsens till eventually a small section of the internal organ pops through.

WHAT TO DO—STRANGULATED HERNIA

SEEK MEDICAL ADVICE. Surgical intervention is usually required.

Touch for Health or One Brain techniques can be helpful in mechanically correcting the problem.

A natural health practitioner will give dietary advice to help avoid aggravation of symptoms.

WHAT TO DO—OTHER HERNIAS

HERBS

The protruding bulge can be gently pushed back and tightly covered with tape under which can be placed a poultice of Comfrey or Hawkweed to help heal the weakened muscle after seeking the advice of a cranial oesteopath or a physiotherapist.

HOMEOPATHIC

Aconite 30c: Vomiting with fear, heat, sweat, and increased urination; intense thirst; bitter taste; burning in region of hernia; hot tense abdomen; sensitive to touch, better from warm drinks, worse at night. Alternate with Nux Vomica at 10–20 minute intervals during acute stages.

Belladonna 30c: Strangulated hernia; bubbling, pulsating bulge, transverse colon protrudes: hot, tender, swollen abdomen. Empty retching; spasms worse from coughing, sneezing, or touch; better from being semi-erect.

Calc Carb 30c: Umbilical or inguinal hernia. Stomach is sensitive to slightest pressure. Cutting pain with sour belching and vomiting.

Lycopodium 30c: Umbilical hernia; thin, withered, full of gas, pressure in stomach with feeling of fullness after slightest food; feeling of fermentation, worse from warm food and drink.

Nux Vomica 30c: Pressing pain from stomach up into chest; Nausea, weight, and pain in stomach; umbilical, hiatus, or strangulated hernia; pressure of a stone several hours after eating; difficult belching; colic with short breath, desire to vomit and pass bowel movement; constant uneasiness in rectum.

CELL SALTS

Calc Fluor: Helps to tighten the loose muscle and give elasticity to the tissues.

Calc Phos: Helps in union of ruptured tissues. Flatulence and heartburn; pain is worse after eating.

Silica: For cramping pains; swelling of area around hernia; vomiting immediately after food.

SEEK MEDICAL ADVICE:

- If there is intense pain, vomiting, and swelling of the abdomen.
- If symptoms persist for more than 12 hours despite above procedure.

A *strangulated hernia* will usually require surgical treatment.

Hives

Hives (Urticaria) may follow stings, insect bites, or trauma. They may also be due to sensitivity to certain foods or drugs, e.g., shellfish, strawberries, eggs, chocolate, penicillin, or antibiotics. Hives may also be associated with worm infestations.

DESCRIPTION

Extremely itchy, red spots, which can be any size or shape, over a large part of the body, especially the mouth and throat. These spots may become swollen and slightly elevated. Hives fade quickly only to reappear elsewhere.

WHAT TO DO—INTERNAL APPLICATIONS

HERBS

Dandelion, Yarrow, and Golden Seal can be taken internally and also used to bathe and soothe the affected parts.

HOMEOPATHIC

Antim Crud 30c: Burning and itching skin, worse from warmth and heat of bed, worse on cheeks and chin.

Camphor 30c: Hives from eating shellfish.

Candida 30c: When rash appears after penicillin or antibiotics.

Pulsatilla 30c: Worse after eating rich foods, often with diarrhea.

Rhus Tox: 30c: Swollen rash with numerous spots; great itching and tingling.

Urtica Urens 30c: Burning, stinging rash. Intolerable itching. Worse after eating shellfish.

CELL SALTS

Kati Phos: Hives caused by food.

Nat Mur: Hives caused by insect bites.

Nat Phos: Hives that appear when worms are suspected.

WHAT TO DO—EXTERNAL APPLICATIONS

Cell salts can be applied locally to the hives by crushing 3–4 tablets and mixing with half a cup of water.

I

Impetigo/School Sores

A contagious infection of the superficial layers of the skin, may be due to a streptococcal or staphylococcal infection.

DESCRIPTION

Starts as red spots on normal skin (usually around nose and mouth). These progress from watery-looking blisters to pus-filled sores that rupture, discharge, and spread. The broken blisters leave raw skin that then forms a crust.

In babies the impetigo usually develops in areas such as the armpit or groin, and in older children it usually starts on the face near the mouth, nose, or ears.

Impetigo can follow a cold.

It can spread rapidly by direct contact. It is more common in warm weather.

WHAT TO DO—EXTERNAL APPLICATIONS

Do not let child touch spots, as this spreads infection, and scratching may result in septicemia (blood poisoning).

HERBS

- Dab infected sores with alcohol (vodka is satisfactory). This helps to clean and dry out the sores, although it does sting for a moment.
- Remove any soft crusts and apply Calendula ointment often.

- Alternatively, oils of Teatree or Thyme can be applied, directly or diluted (2 drops to 3 tsp. Olive or Soya oil).

WHAT TO DO—INTERNAL APPLICATIONS

As antiseptic: Golden Seat
To purify the blood: Drink Dandelion, Echinacea, or Red Clover
To soothe from the inside out: Slippery Elm

HOMEOPATHIC

Check Remedy Pictures for constitutional type.

Antim Crud 30c: Thick, yellow, spreading crusts; thick, white-coated tongue; worse from bathing.

Arsen Alb 30c: Thin, watery discharge that burns and reddens the skin.

Calc Carb 30c: Eruption oozes a thick, bland discharge. Useful during teething.

Hepar Sulph 30c: Soft crusts with thin, yellow pus; sore and bleeding easily; very red and sensitive to touch; worse from cold air and cold bathing.

Mercurius 30c: Sores affect the deeper skin layers; look ulcerated and bleed.

Rhus Tox 30c: Eruptions in clusters; dark-colored discharge with violent burning and itching, tingling and stinging.

Strep/Staph 200: For recurring impetigo or no reaction to well-chosen remedies. (For 200c potency, see page 13.)

NOTE: If the impetigo does not clear up despite persistent treatments, suspect underlying causes such as scabies or head lice (nits).

Infection

Signs of infection (sepsis) are:

- Pus on the surface of a wound.
- If wound has been healing then becomes painful again and surrounding area becomes swollen, red, and hot.
- Red lines running away from the wound.
- Painful swellings in a place near but away from the wound—usually in armpits or groin on same side as wound.
- Rise in temperature, ill health, and shivering.

WHAT TO DO—INTERNAL APPLICATIONS

HERBS

Attack the problem internally with blood-purifying herbs: Comfrey, Golden Seal, Puha, Burdock, Echinacea, Sarsaparilla. These work well in combination. Use the same mixture to bathe the affected area.

Build up child's immunity quickly with plenty of Vitamins A and C.

WHAT TO DO—EXTERNAL APPLICATIONS

Lavender, Rosemary, Thyme, or Teatree act as antiseptics and can be applied mixed or separately (3 drops to 3 tsp. of Olive or Soya oil) dabbed on the area.

HOMEOPATHIC

Hepar Sulph 30c: Sores are common and skin always seems unhealthy.

Pyrogenium 30c: Poison-looking wounds—injury becomes swollen and discolored.

Silica 30c: Every injury tends to develop pus, and swollen glands often appear.

Calc Sulph: Wounds that don't heal readily or neglected wounds.

Kali Mur: For the first stage of redness or swelling.

Silica: Wound is festering.

FOR REPEATED INFECTIONS

It is important to build up the child's natural immunity. Best herbs for this purpose are those mentioned above, so use these for at least three weeks.

SEEK MEDICAL ADVICE

- If temperature goes up in spite of above procedure.
- Red line does not recede or if it progresses.
- Swollen glands do not recede or if they become painful.

Influenza

A highly infectious disease caused by a number of viruses affecting the upper respiratory tract and the body, acting more widely than the common cold virus.

DESCRIPTION

Begins as a headache, fever (highest on the second day 100.4°F) with sore throat, severe pain in limbs and back. After a few days there is more debilitation with running nose and cough, leaving child depressed, exhausted, uncomfortable, and weary.

Incubation Period: 2–3 days.

Recovery Time: 3–7 days if no complications arise.

Complications: Can arise from lack of attention to the recuperation period when depression, palpitations, and bron-cho-pneumonia can develop.

WHAT TO DO—INTERNAL APPLICATIONS

- Bed rest until temperature returns to normal.
- Plenty of diluted pure fruit juices for a few days to rest the digestive organs.
- Avoid food during acute phase. If especially hungry, then give fresh fruit, slowly adding vegetables and avoiding dairy foods, processed foods, breads, and meats.

HERBS

For Fever: Boneset, Yarrow, or Lemon Balm
For disturbed digestion: Cinnamon or Thyme
To relieve congestion: Echinacea, Garlic, Golden Seal, Cayenne, Ginger
To soothe and calm: Elder

WHAT TO DO—EXTERNAL APPLICATIONS

Peppermint or Teatree oil (3 drops diluted with 2 tsp. Olive oil) can be used as a rub on the sore parts.

HOMEOPATHIC

After suspected contact, see Resistance and Immunity, page 19.

Arsen Alb 30c: Can't bear sight or smell of food; sneezing; thin watery discharge; dry cough; painful chest; burning eyes.
Baptisia 30c: Sore muscles, offensive breath, stool, urine, and/or sweat; sense of suffocation in chest.
Eupatorium Perfoliatum 30c: Great soreness and aching all over body; sore larynx and chest; child holds chest during cough because it hurts so much; also pain in head during cough; runny nose and great thirst.

Euphrasia 30c: If the eyes are very much affected.

Gelsernium 30c: Aching limbs; dull, heavy eyes and head; child is weak, tired, and chilly; bouts of sneezing.

Phosphorus 30c: For debility following influenza.

Pyrogenium 30c: Restless, rapid pulse, sweat but no heat; bed feels too hard.

Rhus Tox 30c: Caused by getting wet and cold; sneezing, bone pains, and depression.

Influenzinum or Bacillinum 200c (Nosode—see page 21): To help clear a severe case or for lingering aftereffects of the disease.

CELL SALTS

After contact: Ferr Phos may help child's resistance when taken four times daily for three days.

Main remedy to take throughout course of illness and in conjunction with other appropriate remedies: Nat Sulph.

Calc Phos: During convalescence and remaining weakness.

Ferr Phos: For early signs, hot/cold fever, headache.

Kali Mur: Sore throat, tired and drained feeling.

Mag Phos: To help reduce aches and pains.

Nat Mur: If child sneezes with watery eyes and nose.

The appropriate cell salts can be alternated if desired, at half-hourly intervals, then two-hourly as symptoms become less severe.

TO BUILD RESISTANCE

To help strengthen the immune system and restore to full health after the disease or vaccination, see page 19.

SEEK MEDICAL HELP

- For a throat swab if pus develops on the tonsils.

See also: **Colds, Coughs, Allergies, Sore Throat, Bronchitis** (influenza fever is normally higher than bronchitis).

J

Jaundice

Jaundice is the term given to the yellow discoloration of the skin and conjunctiva (inside eyelid) caused by an excess of bile pigment in the bloodstream. This yellowish color is the indicating symptom.

TYPES OF JAUNDICE

The abnormal presence of bile in the blood may be caused by:

1. Blockage or interference in the bile ducts (obstructive or cholestatic jaundice): caused by gallstones, drugs, recurrent jaundice in pregnancy, or viral hepatitis (see Hepatitis).

    Signs may be pale stools, dark urine, great weight loss, persistent itching, painful enlarged spleen, enlarged neck glands, cholesterol deposits around eyelids.

2. A disorder of liver function (hepatocellular, infective, or toxic jaundice): the liver cells cannot excrete bilirubin into bile duct for excretion.

    Caused by viral infection transmitted by droplets from mouth or nose; yellow fever; drugs or toxic agents such as phosphorus, arsenic, gold, or chloroform.

    In babies, it may be due to an umbilical infection; in older children, it is usually brought about by chemicals.

    After an incubation period of 4–5 weeks, symptoms of gastric disturbance with vomiting persist for many weeks.

3. Excessive destruction of red blood cells (hemolytic or physiological jaundice): occurring within the first few days of life,

it is seldom a serious problem now. (When due to Rh Factor incompatibility, the infant will be kept in hospital and may need a transfusion. This is rare since 1975.)

Caused by: Breakdown of red blood cells present in the newborn as the lung functions take over from the placenta.

Signs: Yellow discoloration of skin and other tissues (not eyes); bowel movements retain their normal color; this type of jaundice passes off after two weeks without complications.

DESCRIPTION

Progressive signs—urine turns dark yellow, olive, dark brown, or black and leaves a stain on the toilet bowl; bowel movements (stools) are bulky, white or pale yellow, and offensive; slight fever; constipation or diarrhea. Child may be anxious, have discomfort in the liver region (right upper abdomen) with slow pulse, disturbed sleep, and itchy skin.

Tongue is coated white or yellow; bitter taste in mouth.

Whites of eyes, insides of eyelids, roots of nails, face, neck, trunk, and limbs can all be affected. The color varies from the lemon-yellow or daffodil tints of hemolytic jaundice (eyelids and whites are not affected here); the shades of yellow, orange, or dark olive green of obstructive jaundice; to the bright yellow of toxic jaundice.

WHAT TO DO

SEEK MEDICAL ADVICE, The cause needs to be identified.

Also, seek advice from a natural health practitioner. Any treatment can be supported by the following:

- Bed rest in a well-ventilated room.
- In infectious jaundice, avoid contact with others.
- In jaundice of the newborn baby, place a few drops of Wheat Germ oil in a dropper into the mouth once daily until yellowness fades.
- Expose child's skin to sunlight gently.

- Light nourishing diet, avoid fats, fried food, alcohol, and roast foods.
- Drink plenty of fluids: skim milk, juices made from lemon, carrot, apple, beetroot, celery, and grapes mixed with honey, if desired, and taken several times daily for months.
- Raw apples, pears, and grapes.
- Barley Water (1 cup barley simmered with 3 liters water for 3 hours and strained).

HERBS

Many herbs are of benefit to the liver during jaundice and convalescence. Mix any combination of the following and drink small glasses 3–4 times daily: Dandelion, Centaury, Irish Moss, Agrimony, Rosehip, Barberry, Blue Flag, Yellow Dock, Golden Seal, Mandrake, Cascara Sagrada.

HOMEOPATHIC

Medicines with alcohol are best avoided, so use tablets.

Aconite 30c: Fever, restlessness, anxiety, pressure and constriction around liver; white stools; alternately loose stools and constipation.

Arsen Alb 30c: Great exhaustion after slight exertion; low vitality; great thirst; no appetite; vomiting of blood and bile; belching; very irritable stomach, swollen painful liver and spleen, burning pain in rectum and anus. Itchy skin. Disturbed restless sleep.

Chelidonium 30c: For jaundiced babies in first few weeks of life, half-crushed tablet or one drop daily till jaundice fades. Biliousness and jaundice, swelling of liver, chilliness, fever, yellow-coated tongue, bitter taste and craving for acid things; stools yellow, profuse, and loose.

China 30c: Exhaustion from long-standing jaundice; white stools with flatulence; stools soft but difficult to pass; swollen liver and spleen; disturbed anxious sleep; thickly coated dirty tongue.

Hydrastis 30c: Bitter taste, lack of appetite, yellow smelly urine, exhaustion, light-colored stools; slimy, swollen, white tongue. Tender liver, constipation.

Merc Corr 30c: Yellow, white-coated tongue with teeth imprints, foul breath, lost appetite; depressed and low-spirited; clay-colored stools with much straining to pass them; yellow skin over eyes; liver region painful to touch; itching all over.

Merc Dulcis 30c: Jaundice in children with offensive breath; nausea and vomiting; dark tongue; bowel movement with bile, mucous, and blood.

Phosphorus 30c: Marked soreness of liver with jaundice; depressed, easily startled; nervous; grayish-white stools; vomiting; painless, copious debilitating diarrhea, dark urine with sediment; great drowsiness; short naps and frequent wakings. Worse from exertion.

Podophyllum 30c: Alternate diarrhea and constipation; loose and watery or hard and clay-colored stool; yellow face and eyes; vomiting; hot, sour belching; foul taste; liver painful, worse from rubbing; pain under right shoulder blade; white or yellow-coated tongue. Maybe gallstones.

Sulphur 30c: Chronic jaundice though not indicated if stools are colorless. Irritable, depressed, thin and weak with good appetite; itchy skin; sore and red anus; morning diarrhea; wakens suddenly.

NOTE: Cholesterinum 6x—three times daily for 2–4 weeks taken with your choice of above, for burning pain in side, gallstones, hurts so much, holds hands on sides.

CELL SALTS

Ferr Phos: For pain in liver with vomiting of undigested food.

Kali Mur: Jaundice with catarrhal condition; constipation; light-colored stools.

Kali Sulph: Slimy-yellow coating on tongue, catarrh of stomach; fullness at pit of stomach.

Nat Mur: Jaundice associated with drowsiness, watery secretions, thirst, dryness of skin.

See also: **Hepatitis**.

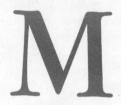

Measles

An infectious disease

A highly contagious viral infection transferred by droplets from the mouth or nose when child coughs, talks, or sneezes.

DESCRIPTION

Begins with cold symptoms—runny nose, sore throat, cough, red watery eyes, often a dislike of bright light and a fever that becomes progressively higher (up to 105°F). About four days later, a rash of red-pink blotches appear—first behind the ears and on the face, sometimes inside the mouth, and spreading to trunk and limbs. The fever should subside at this stage. After another 5–7 days the rash begins to fade. The fever accompanying measles can become very high, and the appetite may be completely lost.

Most common age: 8 months to 5 years.
Incubation period: 10–14 days.
Isolation period: 1 week after rash appears.
Recovery time: A mild attack is over well within a fortnight.
Complications: Secondary infection of middle ear, throat, larynx, or lungs; encephalitis; visual disturbances.

WHAT TO DO

- Put to bed and avoid bright lights.
- Keep out those visitors who have colds and sore throats.

- Have room quiet and warm.
- Avoid use of eyes, e.g., reading or watching television.
- Drink lots of fluids; if child has no appetite, he/she will receive adequate nourishment from herb teas and diluted fruit or vegetable juices during the acute stage of the illness.
- If earache develops, seek professional advice from your doctor or homeopath.

SEEK MEDICAL ADVICE if signs of pneumonia, meningitis, severe tummy pain develop.

HERBS

For cough: Mullein
For fever: Boneset
For restoring energy: Gentian
To calm and soothe the system: Hops or Elder
To ease the rash: Red Clover
To move the bowels: Licorice
To provide extra nourishment during illness: Lavender, Teatree, or Thyme

Inhalation:
Oils of Lavender (3 drops), Teatree (2 drops), and Thyme (1 drop) mixed with steaming water (4¼ cups) can be breathed in to help the nose and eyes.

External:
Thyme oil (3 drops) can be mixed with Olive or Soya oil (2 tsp.) and rubbed on rash to soothe.

HOMEOPATHIC

After suspected contact, see Resistance and Immunity, page 19.

Apis 30c: High temperature, very hot and wanting covers off, sore eyes, tearful and irritable.
Bryonia 30c: Tiresome cough. High temperature, swollen face

with dull look, complains of headache, intense thirst for cold water, feels chilly but wants air. Dry, hard, painful cough; appearance of rash is delayed.

Euphrasia 30c: Red, swollen eyelids and great sensitivity to light.

Gelsemium 30c: Very high fever, limbs feel too heavy to move; maybe delirium. Harsh, barking cough with sore chest and dislike of company. Absence of thirst with dry tongue; red, itchy skin.

Phosphorus 30c: Chest symptoms prominent; troublesome dry cough and tightness in chest; thirst for cold water, which may be vomited.

Pulsatilla 30c: Useful after fever stage. Very restless and irritable, wants to be constantly waited on; child must sit up with troublesome cough, loose by day and dry by night; maybe nausea, diarrhea, or earache.

Morbillinum 200c (Nosode—see page 21): To help clear a severe case or for lingering aftereffects of the disease. Do not give while disease is incubating.

CELL SALTS

Ferr Phos: First remedy for fever and until eruption appears.

Kali Mur: Coated tongue, ear problems, swollen glands, and hoarse cough.

Nat Mur: Very itchy skin and watery nose and eyes.

Give the appropriate cell salt hourly until the eruption appears. They may be alternated if necessary. Alternate Calc Phos and Kali Sulph during the final stages to help clear the condition and restore energy.

TO BUILD RESISTANCE

To help strengthen the immune system and restore to full health after the disease (or vaccination), see page 19.

SEEK MEDICAL ADVICE if child develops:

- Shortness of breath with the cough
- Earache or swollen glands
- Convulsions
- Headache and vomiting
- Lethargy and lack of awareness of surroundings
- Eyes become stuck together and very red
- Fever *remains* two days after the spots appear
- Severe tummy pain

See also: Rubella, Scarlet Fever, Bronchitis, Influenza.

Meningitis

A notifiable disease. Must be reported immediately to your doctor or local Health Department.

Inflammation of the meninges (brain lining) caused by bacterial, chemical, fungal, or viral invasion.

Meningitis can be epidemic or follow an infection, e.g., respiratory, middle ear, or sinus.

DESCRIPTION

Some or all of the following may occur: fever and stiff neck, headache, irritable and drowsy; can deteriorate to include convulsions, delirium, and respiratory difficulties.

Incubation period: 3–7 days.
Isolation period: until cured.
Complications: hydrocephalus, nerve palsy, renal failure.

WHAT TO DO

SEEK MEDICAL ADVICE IMMEDIATELY. Successful recovery depends on speed of treatment. Child will be admitted to hospital for lumbar puncture and blood tests and probably get intravenous antibiotics.

The following procedure is included for your information to aid in restoring to full health after medical treatment or until medical aid arrives. Take child off all foods and give a diet of fresh fruit juices and vegetable juices, herb teas, and broths.

HERBS

Combine any of the following:

To calm the nervous system: Skullcap or Valerian
To fight the infection: Golden Seal
To provide extra nourishment during the illness: Peppermint and Rosemary
To reduce fever: Yarrow

HOMEOPATHIC

After suspected contact, see Resistance and Immunity, page 19.

Aconite 30c: Useful at beginning when fear is marked. If symptoms come on after exposure to the sun.

Apis 30c: Shrill outcries in sleep; fidgety; violent fever, swelling and grinding of teeth.

Belladonna 30c: Burning fever; throat spasm worse from swallowing; uncontrollable vomiting; bluish-red facial color; dilated eyes; headache. Worse from light noise and jarring. Starts in sleep and grinds teeth. Violent symptoms.

Bryonia 30c: Chewing motion of mouth; screams with pain if moved; distended abdomen; copious sweat; drinks in greedy fashion. Face flushes and pales alternately. White tongue.

Calc Carb 30c: Large-headed children; pale face; large abdomen; sweaty head worse during sleep; screaming without cause, strong urine.

Cuprum 30c: Excessive vomiting, worse from movement or touch; convulsions with blue face and contracted jaws; craves cold water. Violent delirium, rolling eyeballs, deep sleep.

Helleborus 30c: Unconscious moaning, rolling head, dropping jaw; foul smell; cannot be fully aroused; wrinkling of forehead; automatic movements of one arm and leg. Eyeballs turned upward, shooting pains in head, bores head into pillow.

Stramonium 30c: Convulsions of upper extremities and isolated muscles; staggering, stammering, vomiting green bile; terrified expression; cannot swallow because of spasm.

Zincum 30c: Sharp pains in head; fidgety feet; little or no fever. Hypersensitivity of skin and senses.

Meningococcin 200c (Nosode—see page 21): To help clear a severe case or for lingering aftereffects of the disease. *Do not give while disease is incubating.*

CELL SALTS

All of the following are needed: Ferr Phos and Kali Phos to be alternated every half-hour. Nat Mur: Give this also at two-hourly intervals. Silica: Give this once daily.

TO BUILD RESISTANCE

To help strengthen the immune system, restore to full health after the disease (or vaccination), see Resistance and Immunity, page 19.

Menstruation

The appearance of the first menstrual period varies from ages 9–18, but is most common between ages 12–14.

For some girls approaching their teenage years, the hormonal changes can cause major discomfort in the form of mood changes, period pains, heavy or irregular periods, headaches, fevers, nausea, dizziness, or vomiting.

These symptoms can serve a useful purpose by showing us the constitutional tendencies of the person concerned. Homeopathy and herbs have much to offer for this issue. We feel that by dealing with these crises when they first occur, many potential adult problems can be avoided.

WHAT TO DO

The remedies below may not offer a solution for every young woman, in which case we recommend that you seek expert herbal or homeopathic advice.

For the emotional problems associated with hormonal changes, Bach Flower Essences have much to offer. Related books and remedies are available from most health shops.

HERBS

For an irregular cycle or absent period (unless pregnancy is suspected): Blue Cohosh, False Unicorn Rt, Sabina, Rue, Southernwood, Tansy, Pennyroyal, Parsley, Senecio, Motherwort, Black Cohosh, Blessed Thistle, or Vitex Agnus Castus

Heavy flow: Ladies Mantle, Plantain, Comfrey, Mistletoe, Blessed Thistle, Yarrow, Don Quai

Painful cramps: Cramp Bark, Passionflower, Black Cohosh, False Unicorn Rt, Wild Yam, Dandelion, Chamomile

Premenstrual tension: Scullcap, Valerian, Chamomile, Bach Flower Essences

HOMEOPATHY

Aconite 30c: Period suppressed due to chill or fright; headache with apprehension and restlessness. Worse from heat. Thirsty with red face.

Belladonna 30c: Irregular and profuse. Face red and flushed, thirsty, restless, and irritable. Cutting pains.

Bryonia 30c: Irregular or suppressed period with headache or nosebleed, and constipation.

Calc Carb 30c: First period begins very early. Sluggish, overweight, and pale; itchy genitals before period with tender, swollen breasts. Headache, colic, chilliness and sweat are common before the period.

Calc Phos 30c: Early and heavy period with backache, worse from exposure to cold and damp weather.

Chamomile 30c: Severe colicky pains, restless and irritable, diarrhea and fainting.

Ferr Met 30c: Thin, tired, anemic girl with irregular period of pale watery blood.

Graphites 30c: Very late first period. Irregular period with constipation, itching of genitals, swollen, hard breasts, and skin problems.

Ignatia 30c: Period is affected by grief or shock.

Kali Carb 30c: Delayed and difficult first period in young girls accompanied by fear and anxiety and pain through back, abdomen, and genitals.

Nat Mur 30c: Early, heavy period in a weepy, emotional girl with shiny facial skin.

Nux Vomica 30c: Painful cramps and violent spasms, irritable and constipated.

Pulsatilla 30c: First period is delayed, slight loss only, with back pain, nausea, crying, vomiting. Period is changeable, may stop suddenly after exposure to dampness or wet.

Sepia 30c: Depressed, irritable and solitary girl; thin, tired, sallow-colored skin, dragging down pains in abdomen; frequently delayed period.

Sulphur 30c: Untidy, disorganized person. Hot, burning period pains; red face, bloody nose, irregular period stopping suddenly or preceded by headache.

CELL SALTS

Calc Phos: Scanty flow, difficult first periods, anemic with colicky pains and backache.

Ferr Phos: Painful period preceded by congestion in pelvic organs and headache. Flushing, fever, and vomiting.

Kali Mur: Painful period worse from taking cold; blood is a

very dark color.

Kali Phos: Menstrual colic in pale, tearful, irritable, sensitive, nervous girls.

Mag Phos: Spasms of cramplike pain in lower abdomen causing her to bend over double; better from heat and movement.

Nat Mur: Irregular period, scanty and dark, preceded by frontal headache, flow is irritating; girl is depressed and withdrawn.

Silica: Icy coldness of entire body before and during period with constipation, anxiety, and oversensitive nature.

Mouth Ulcers

Recurrent, painful mouth sores. If one or more sores causes bleeding when scraped, thrush is suspected. Cracks at corners of mouth indicate Vitamin B_2 or B_3 deficiency. Nuts, chocolates, and citrus fruits can cause recurrence of mouth ulcers; ulcers may also be caused by bowel inflammation or physical and emotional stress.

WHAT TO DO

HERBS

Gargle and also use as herbal tea one or more of the following herbs: Myrrh, Golden Seal, Raspberry, Marjoram, or Sage. Teatree oil may be applied directly to the ulcer.

HOMEOPATHIC

Borax 30c: Small ulcers that bleed if touched, or when eating; mouth is hot.

Mercurius 30c: Much saliva with spongy gums, sweet metallic taste and thirst.

Nitric Acid 30c: Ulcers with splinterlike pains, bad breath, and much saliva. Whitish gums.

Calc Phos: Blisters on tip of tongue; cold sores or chapped lips.
Kali Mur: Rawness of mouth.
Nat Mur: Blisters on tongue.
Silica: Ulcers on tongue.
See also: **Thrush, p. 213, Cold Sores, p. 75.**

Mumps

An infectious disease.
A viral infection of one or both parotid glands.

The virus spreads by means of droplets from the mouth or nose while coughing, talking, or sneezing.

DESCRIPTION

Begins with nasal catarrh, a rise in temperature (99.5–103°F), a mild feeling of illness, and tenderness around the ears, followed by swelling of the parotid gland (situated immediately in front of the ear lobes and at the angle of the jaw). The other parotid usually swells a day or two later. There is pain on chewing and opening mouth and the outline of the face is altered considerably.

Note: Swelling is particularly in front, below and behind the ear lobe and when swollen, is hard, tense, and immovable. If there is any doubt, seek further advice in order to distinguish from the more serious diphtheria. (However, this is no longer common.)

Most common age: 5 to 15 years.
Incubation period: 18 days.
Isolation period: For 9 days from the date of onset or until swelling of all involved glands has completely subsided and the patient has returned to normal.
Recovery time: 7–10 days.

WHAT TO DO

- Rest and warmth.
- Restricted diet of fresh fruits, vegetables, soups, broths, and fresh juices.

HERBS

Daily drinks of Red Clover tea during the mumps and afterward to clear out the lymph glands.

Keep bowels clear by drinking Licorice and Rosemary tea.

HOMEOPATHIC

After suspected contact: Pilocarpine 30c. This can help the child's resistance to the disease. Give one dose night and morning for three days (starting within 2 days of contact), then one dose per week for 2 weeks.

Belladonna 30c: Bright red swelling on right side; also useful where swelling disappears and head or neck pain develops.

Bryonia 30c: Hard swelling with tenderness; slightest motion of head is painful; irritable; dry lips; very thirsty for large quantities of water.

Mercurius 30c: For slight fever with tenderness in neck area; excess saliva and offensive breath; much pain and stiffness in jaws.

Pulsatilla 30c: If disease lingers, weepy, whining, thirstless child who craves the open air.

Rhus Tox 30c: Dark, red swellings; sticking pains on swallowing; worse left side.

Parotidinum 200c (Nosode—see page 21): To help clear a severe case, or for lingering aftereffects of the disease. *Do not give while disease is incubating.*

Calc Fluor: If swelling persists past expected duration.

Ferr Phos: For early stage of fever and pain.

Kali Mur and Nat Mur: Alternate when gland is swollen and painful with thickly-coated white tongue.

SEEK MEDICAL ADVICE

- If the child develops a bad headache, vomiting, neck stiffness, or drowsiness
- If boys of eleven years or older develop swelling and pain in the testicles
- If girls of eleven years or older develop breast pains
- If any other glands are swollen

TO BUILD RESISTANCE

To strengthen the immune system and to help restore to full health after the disease or the vaccination, see Resistance and Immunity, page 19.

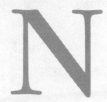

Nose

1 Congestion
2 Nosebleed
3 Object in the nose

1 Congestion

Congestion can involve a blocked nose, a free-flowing discharge, or a thick, yellow discharge (which often indicates infection).

It can also coincide with influenza, measles, colds, or allergies. See also: **Sinusitis.**

WHAT TO DO

HERBS

For Vitamin C: Rosehip
To cleanse: Thyme
To dry up mucous: Yarrow
To provide extra nourishment: Clove, Aniseed, or Thyme
To soothe the mucous membranes: Slippery Elm

Mix any of these together and drink warm throughout the day.
Inhalation: To clear nostrils: 3–8 drops of Thyme, Peppermint, or Teatree oil into a basin of steaming water. Place head over basin, cover head with towel, and breathe in the vapor for ten minutes.

Repeat as required.

HOMEOPATHIC

Aconite 30c: Nose is swollen, dry, or blocked with tingling, burning, and throbbing sensations. Worse from cold, dry winds, better in open air.

Arsen Alb 30c: Thin, watery discharge that burns the skin; intense tickling; nose feels blocked. Chilliness, sneezing. Worse in open air.

Gelsemium 30c: Sneezing, runny nose with heavy eyes, fullness at root of nose, headache; child is worse in warm weather.

Hepar Sulph 30c: Nose is blocked in cold air; discharge becomes thick, yellow; nose is painful and swollen; child is irritable. Easy recurrence accompanied by sticking in throat.

Mercurius 30c: Nostrils are raw and ulcerated with thin mucous, burning in eyes and nose; frontal sinus involvement.

Nat Mur 30c: For colds beginning with a sneeze; watery, clear discharge; loss of smell and taste. Blisters around mouth and nose.

Nux Vomica 30c: Nose is alternately dry and runny in the daytime, blocked at night and outdoors.

Pulsatilla 30c: Thick, yellow, bland discharge; loss of taste, smell and appetite; better in the cool air; worse from warmth.

CELL SALTS

Calc Phos: Swollen, ulcerated nostrils; icy cold tip of nose; child takes cold easily.

Kali Mur: Discharge drops down back of throat; or is thick and white. Kali Sulph: Yellow, slimy discharge.

Nat Mur: Thin, salty, watery discharge; sneezing.

Nat Sulph: Discharge is either green and profuse or dry and burning.

Silica: Nostrils are either red and sore or itchy and dry.

FOR RECURRING CONGESTION

Refer to Allergies if nasal congestion often recurs. Incompletely cleared infections may contribute to nasal congestion.

Homeopathic: Strep/Staph 200c can help to clear this problem. (For 200c potency, see page 13).

Herbal: Rosehip, Echinacea, Golden Seal, and Mullein can be taken daily for several weeks. These are rich in Vitamins A and C, which help fight infection.

2 Nosebleed

Sit child up, leaning forward with a pad to collect blood. (Swallowing the blood can interfere with clotting, so if a child continues to swallow, a cork held between their teeth can help to stop this.) Squeeze the soft part of the nose at nostrils for ten minutes by the clock. Release and observe—if bleeding continues, repeat. Don't let child blow his/her nose for several hours.

Externally: Cold water or ice can be applied to the root of the nose to stop bleeding.

HERBS

Yarrow or Plantain tea sipped at 15–minute intervals.

Hamamelis tincture (10 drops in half-cup water) can be used as nose drops (1 drop to each nostril at 5–minute intervals), and can also be taken internally (five drops at 15–minute intervals).

HOMEOPATHIC

Aconite 30c: Bright, red-colored blood; child may be anxious or feverish.

Arnica 30c: If bleeding is result of injury.

Hamamelis 30c: Profuse bleeding from nose, noncoagulating flow.

Arsen Album 30c: For recurrent nosebleeds with burning pains and irritability.

China 30c: Easy bleeding from nose, worse after rising and after heavy blowing of nose. Paleness, fainting in anemic children.

Millefolium 30c: Bright red discharge, maybe after injury. No anxiety.

CELL SALTS

Mix Ferr Phos and Kali Mur, three tablets of each mixed in a cup of water and sipped every few minutes during nosebleed.

If tendency is common, take these cell salts twice daily for three weeks.

3 Object in the nose

Child may have difficulty breathing through nose; nose may appear swollen; blood-stained discharge may be seen.

WHAT TO DO

SEEK MEDICAL OR HOSPITAL AID

- If object is sharp. Do not attempt to remove the object as it may cause damage to nasal tissues. Advise child to breathe through mouth in the meantime.
- If object is hard or spherical (e.g., a marble) as it may go in further. There is then danger of the object going into the lungs or blocking the airways. Advise child to breathe through mouth and do not attempt to remove object.
- If object is visible and soft, have child blow out blocked side twice. If it doesn't come out, seek medical or hospital aid.

P

Pain

Pain is nature's warning that there is a disease process happening. Pain is the message provided by nerves that are present in all body tissue.

It is not always wise to kill pain. Instead, try to find ways to assist the body's natural healing process.

WHAT TO DO

HERBS

Colic pains: Peppermint or Aniseed
Digestive pain: Meadowsweet, Ginger, or Valerian
For kidney or bladder pain: Uva Ursi
Pain of swollen glands: Poke Root or Sassafras
To calm the nervous system: Lobelia, Jamaica Dogwood, Hops, or Valerian

HOMEOPATHIC

Aconite 30c: Pain of toothache and ears; anxious, restless child.
Belladonna 30c: Hot, throbbing pains.
Chamomilla 30c: Intolerable pains, child cries and moans a lot.
Colocynth 30c: Stomach pains, colic, better from bending double.
Hypericum 30c: Pain in damaged nerves.
Rhus Tox 30c: Pain in damaged muscles and ligaments.

Ruta Grav 30c: Pain in damaged bones or old sprains.

Staphysagria 30c: Lingering pain after surgical operations.

CELL SALTS

Ferr Phos: Throbbing, inflammation, pain in back of head; sprains, strains, cuts, and wounds (crushed tablet mixed with a little water can be applied externally on wounds, cuts, sprains, or strains).

Kali Mur: Gastric pain after fatty rich food; white tongue worse moving; dull, aching muscular pains or swellings.

Kali Sulph: Shifting pains, pressure and fullness in stomach, worse outdoors.

Mag Phos: Frontal headache; colic or flatulence, gripes, indigestion, stabbing, boring or shooting pains.

Silica: Pains of boils and abscesses.

CHRONIC PAIN

Some people suffer from long-standing or frequently recurring pain as a result of old injuries (such as broken bones) or past illnesses (such as rheumatic fever). SEEK ADVICE from a homeopath or a Touch for Health instructor.

Pneumonia

Pneumonia is an inflammation of the lung, caused by invasion of the pneumonia germ or other germs or viruses. Fluid fills up the lung spaces, making oxygenation less efficient.

DESCRIPTION

Usually starts as a cold with a high fever (103–105.8°F), chills, nausea, severe pain in chest usually on one side, coughing up rusty-colored, yellow or greenish mucous.

Rapid, shallow breathing; face or fingertips become blue from lack of oxygen; tongue is furred. (Do not confuse with rapid *deep* breathing of dehydration or hyperventilation.)

WHAT TO DO

SEEK MEDICAL ADVICE IMMEDIATELY

Most children with pneumonia will need antibiotics. The following procedures can be used until medical aid arrives or to help restore child to full health *after medical treatment*.

To aid recovery: Plenty of fluid in the form of fresh fruit or vegetable juices, water, or broths. Avoid dairy foods, wheat products, all forms of sugar and sweetened products.

Inhalation: Oils of Lemon, Lavender, Teatree, or Juniper (1 drop of each is usually sufficient) can be added to steaming water and breathed in.

HERBS

Make a mixture from the following:

To cleanse and purify blood: Golden Seal or Garlic
To ease chest pain: Marshmallow or Mullein
To move the bowels and thus help eliminate toxins: Licorice or Rosemary
To provide extra nourishment during the illness: Lemon, Lavender, Teatree, and/or Juniper

External: Applications to the chest are very soothing, especially to help through the night. Slightly warm the following mixture and rub onto chest at night and during the day if needed: 2 drops each of Lavender, Lemon, Juniper, and Teatree (or Eucalyptus) oils mixed with 2 Tbs. Olive, Soya, or Almond oil.

HOMEOPATHIC

Aconite 30c: Early stage for strong children in whom the attack is sudden; due to cold, dry winds; high sudden fever, hoarse dry cough, short breath, anxiety, palpitations; frothy, watery, or blood-tinged sputum; very restless.

Antim Tart 30c: Difficult breathing, worse toward morning, worse from lying down; sharp, burning pains with high fever and occasional vomiting; difficult to raise mucous despite great rattling in chest.

Bryonia 30c: Child lies quietly, cough is dry and painful with scanty rust-colored sputum. Better from lying on painful or right side, and from keeping still. Child holds breath for fear of cough being too painful.

Iodum 30c: Restlessness with high fever, great difficulty in breathing; blood-streaked sputum, internal heat while externally cold. There may be no pain.

Phosphorus 30c: Pneumonia may come on after measles; hot, tight, painful chest; rattling of mucous with yellow, rusty, or blood-streaked sputum. Whole body trembles with the cough. Child is better with sleep and darkness. Feeling of a great load on chest.

Sulphur 30c: Rattling in chest, thick yellow/green sputum, dry tongue, fever; no improvement from other remedies.

Pneumococcin 200c (Nosode—see page 21): To help clear a severe case or for lingering aftereffects of the disease. *Do not give while disease is incubating.*

CELL SALTS

Ferr Phos: During initial stages of infection; short, painful cough; hot chest.

Kali Mur: Thick, white expectoration. Rattling chest.

Kali Sulph: Yellow, slimy, sticky, or green mucous; great rattling and wheezing, better in cool air.

LONG-TERM SUPPORT

- Depending on the type of pneumonia, specific homeopathic Nosodes are available to help clear residual poisons and restore to full health. Particular homeopathic remedies that may be found useful are Streptococcin, Influenzinum, Bacillinum, and Pneumococcin. Seek homeopathic advice for use of these.

- After such a debilitating illness, herbal tonics will help to strengthen the vitality of the lungs and the system in general. These should be continued for several months: Gentian, Mullein, Lungwort, Chamomile, Burdock, and Elecampane.

Poisoning

Ingested Poison—Type 1
Ingested Poison—Type 2

1. IMMEDIATE TREATMENT IS ESSENTIAL FOR ALL POISONS.
2. DO NOT INDUCE VOMITING UNTIL POISON HAS BEEN IDENTIFIED. SEE BELOW.

    If lips or mouth show signs of burning, cool by giving water or milk to drink.

    If unconscious or convulsing, place gently on side with head sideways in recovery position to clear airways and prevent choking. *Do not give fluids. Do not induce vomiting.*

    If breathing or heartbeat have stopped, begin resuscitation immediately. *Take care not to contaminate yourself* with poison that may be around the child's mouth.
3. IF SERIOUS, CALL AN AMBULANCE.

    Collect samples of vomit and containers such as bottles, etc. If you know what poison your child took, see below.

Note: Poisoning must be treated seriously. Although the treatments below are a useful follow-up, it is advisable to seek medical advice as well.

Ingested Poison—Type 1

Aspirin, drugs, chemicals, poisonous plants, alcohol, rat poison, match boxes, methylated spirits, disinfectants (except those containing pine or lavender).

DESCRIPTION

Vomiting, nausea, delirium, cramps, rapid pulse, abdominal pain, drowsiness, hot flushed skin, blurred vision, sweating.

WHAT TO DO

1. Give at least one glass of milk immediately.
2. Induce vomiting in *one* of the following ways:

   - Putting fingers down throat
   - Syrup of Ipecac (dosage: 3 tsp. for one-year-old; 5 tsp. for three-year-old; 6 tsp. for older children; 3 Tbs. for adults)
   - 1 Tbs. salt to half a glass of warm water. Make child gulp this down quickly. Continue until child has vomited at least twice. (Exception: For poisonous mushrooms, mix instead 1 Tbs. of dry mustard.)

3. Give charcoal to absorb residual poisons.
4. SEEK MEDICAL ADVICE, taking with you a sample of poison or container, and a sample of vomit if possible.

Ingested Poison—Type 2

Corrosive acids, alkalis, detergents, disinfectants containing pine or lavender, ammonia, bleaches, caustic soda, insecticides containing kerosene or petrol, kerosene, turpentine, petroleum products.

DESCRIPTION

Burns to lips, mouth, throat, and stomach; cold, clammy skin, collapse, intense pain.

WHAT TO DO

1. *Do not induce vomiting.*

2. Give fruit juice and water (or milk and water) and follow with beaten egg whites.
3. SEEK MEDICAL ADVICE, taking a sample of vomit (if child has already vomited) and poison to hospital or nearest doctor, if there is no hospital nearby.

POISON ON SKIN

This shows as lumps, rash, and itching (or stinging—blistering and peeling may develop).

WHAT TO DO

1. Remove chemical quickly but be cautious for your own safety.
2. Wash skin thoroughly with water for at least 10 minutes.
3. Remove clothing while flooding the injured part. Then keep cool with wet flannel.
4. SEEK MEDICAL ADVICE. If industrial poison, remove clothes and wash child thoroughly with water.

POISON IN EYES

Signs may be pain, watering, swelling, redness, or spasm.

WHAT TO DO

1. TAKE IMMEDIATE ACTION. Open eyelids and flush freely with cold water, being sure to spray under the lids (e.g., if the eye is shut in a spasm, pull the lids open gently but firmly).
2. Continue until relief is obtained, then cover with eye pad.
3. SEEK MEDICAL AID.

FOOD POISONING

Pain, nausea, vomiting, and diarrhea present within twenty-four hours of consumption of suspected spoiled food. See Internal Approach below.

INHALED POISONS

Signs may be: difficult breathing, lightheadedness, and dizziness; blueness of eyes, nose, fingers, toes, or lips; convulsions.

WHAT TO DO

Protect yourself. Take child into fresh air and encourage deep breathing. If child is not breathing, but you can feel a pulse, loosen clothing and apply mouth-to-mouth resuscitation (unless poisoning is from industrial gases). See Emergency Techniques, page 108, until medical help arrives.

INTERNAL APPROACH FOR ALL POISONINGS

HERBS

To help eliminate poisons, have child drink the following herbs for several weeks following poisoning: Red Clover, Golden Seal, Dandelion, Echinacea, Myrrh, Licorice Root, Barberry, and Capsicum.

HOMEOPATHIC

Aconite 30c: Restless and tossing with great fear and anxiety.

Arsen Alb 30c: Severe vomiting and purging, extreme exhaustion and restlessness; food poisoning.

Cantharis 30c: Fiery burning sensations, burning urine, and pale face.

Carbo Veg 30c: Deathly cold but feels hot inside; better from belching; stomach pain; food poisoning.

Veratrum Alb 30c: Severe vomiting and purging, extreme exhaustion, cold sweat on brow and collapse.

CELL SALTS

Calc Phos: Blisters and swelling on tongue.

Ferr Phos: For congestion with throbbing pulse and burning skin, throat, or stomach.

Kali Phos and Mag Phos for convulsions, or shortness of breath.

Kali Sulph: Dry, hot, and burning in stomach and on skin.

Nat Phos: Nausea, vomiting, and pain, acid taste in mouth.

Many poisons can be antidoted. Always seek further advice from a competent homeopath or medical doctor

Poison Control Center: (800)764-7661 or call (202)362-7217 to find the poison control center nearest you.

See: **Bites & Stings, page 53, for Poisonous Creatures**.

Poliomyelitis

A notifiable disease. Must be reported to your medical doctor or local health department.

A viral infection that enters through the nose and causes inflammation of the spinal cord.

DESCRIPTION

Very sudden onset; general sickness, fever, and headache; maybe vomiting and diarrhea, depression, pain in limbs, and sore throat.

Small proportion of those affected develop paralysis, which progresses rapidly over a few days.

Isolation period: For seven days from the date of onset of the disease, and until fever subsides.

Incubation: Two weeks.

Complications: Permanent paralysis or impairment of mobility, death from paralysis of breathing passages.

WHAT TO DO

SEEK MEDICAL ADVICE IMMEDIATELY.

The following procedures can be helpful in aiding the return to full health *after medical treatment or until medical aid arrives.* Be thoroughly hygienic with kitchen and toilet habits.

HERBS

To help calm, soothe, and cleanse the system during the infection: Sage, Rosemary, Mint, and Lavender can be sipped often throughout the day.

HOMEOPATHIC

After suspected contact, see Resistance and Immunity, page 19.

Causticum 30c: For dry, hoarse cough, dry throat, indistinct speech; paralysis of single parts.

Gelsemium 30c: For great fear, nervous anticipation with trembling and lethargy; aching pain in limbs; chilly with heavy head and dusky-red face.

Lathyrus 30c: Weakness and heaviness; slow recovery of nerve power; numbness, tingling, and paralysis.

Polio 200c (Nosode—see page 21): To help clear a severe case or for lingering aftereffects of the disease. Do *not give while disease is incubating.*

CELL SALTS

Kali Phos needs to be given every two hours during acute phase, then every four hours until symptoms have passed.

TO BUILD RESISTANCE

To help strengthen the immune system and restore to full health after the disease (or vaccination), see Resistance and Immunity, page 19.

Psoriasis

An acute or chronic inflammatory skin disease often inherited. Metabolic disturbances are common, specifically in the small intestine where fat is improperly metabolized.

DESCRIPTION

A thick layer of whitish or silvery scales, usually on knees, elbows, scalp, and trunk. May also be on nails, palms, and soles. Itching is mild, if any. There may be reddened areas of skin. Scratching causes bleeding, but there is no flow of fluid such as occurs in eczema.

WHAT TO DO

- Avoid refined, processed foods, soap, sugar, and sugar products, fatty foods, eggs, dairy products, citrus fruit, and citrus juice.
- Expose skin to sunshine, seawater, or salt baths once weekly; or a half-cup cider vinegar in bathwater to restore acidity.
- 2–3 drops of Lavender oil can be added to bathwater.
- Wash hair with Jojoba shampoo and rinse with a half-cup cider vinegar to 1 liter water.
- Good foods to eat: carrot, beetroot, cucumber, grape, sesame seed and sesame oil.

HERBS

Internally: To purify the blood, stimulate the liver, and help metabolic processes, combine any of the following and drink regularly for three weeks, stop for one week, then repeat: Burdock, Dandelion, Sassafras Red Clover, Slippery Elm, and Valerian.

Externally: Marshmallow or Comfrey ointment can be helpful.

HOMEOPATHIC

We advise that you seek the help of an experienced natural health practitioner. Natural remedies can offer significant help to sufferers of psoriasis.

Arsen Alb 30c: Thickened skin that burns, itches, and swells.

Graphites 30c: Eruptions worse behind ears, palms or backs of hands, bends of joints and folds of skin.

Kali Brom 30c: A leading remedy especially if child is the nervous type, and no clear symptoms arise.

Lycopodium 30c: Dry, withered, scaly eruptions.

Petroleum 30c: Rough, cracked, and leathery; itchy, worse on hands and in cold weather.

Sulphur 30c: Dry, scaly, unhealthy skin; heat and itching of scalp, which is dry and worse from washing.

Tuberculinum 30c: Chronic psoriasis, especially with family history of TB.

CELL SALTS

Calc *Fluor:* For thick, tough, cracked skin.

Calc *Phos:* For red, itchy skin.

Kali Phos: *For* nervous child.

Kali Sulph: *For peeling* skin.

These can be *combined* favorably and taken daily for at least three weeks, stop for *one* week, and repeat if necessary.

Rheumatic Fever

Believed to be a long-term complication from streptococcus A-type infections. Inflammation of the connective tissue in joints, heart, and blood vessels.

Complications: Bronchopneumonia, pleurisy, chorea (involuntary flicking movements), skin eruptions, heart disorders such as change in normal rhythm of heartbeats, heart murmurs (due to heart valve damage), galloping heart tones, heart failure.

DESCRIPTION

May be sudden onset of pain and stiffness in one or more joints; often moving to other joints; sweating; fever; rapid heartbeats; appetite loss.

May be slow onset with fatigue, general ill health, and weight loss. May be increased number of white blood cells.

WHAT TO DO—INTERNAL APPLICATION

SEEK MEDICAL ADVICE

- Because of complications, place child under the care of experts in the medical and natural health field. (A throat culture is essential.) Bed rest, calm, and a stress-free environment are needed. Give a liquid diet initially—plenty of fluid—apple juice or apple cider vinegar/water.

- Later add citrus fruits, greens, and root vegetables, fish, and white meats.
- Avoid meat, egg, dairy products, pickles, refined carbohydrates, sugar and spices, rhubarb, gooseberries, coffee, and tea.
- *Massage* helps stimulate circulation to the affected parts and prevents toxic deposits from settling in joints.

HERBS

For pain: Lobelia

To help remove stress and calm the heart especially: Skullcap, Passionflower, Hawthorn, Valerian, Mistletoe, or Motherwort

To induce sweating and lower fever: Yarrow, Elder, Peppermint, or Pleurisy Root

To stimulate appetite and remove fatigue: Ginger, Gentian

WHAT TO DO—EXTERNAL APPLICATION

Lavender, Peppermint, and/or Rosemary oils can be rubbed on to the skin at site of painful joints. Mix 2–3 drops with 2–3 tsp. Soya or Almond oil and massage.

Lobelia and Hypericum tinctures can also be rubbed on to affected parts.

HOMEOPATHIC

Aconite 30c: Restless and thirsty with fever and dry, hot skin. Scanty urine, stitching pain in chest, hot, pale or red swelling of joints, restless and shifting from one place to another.

Belladonna 30c: High fever, joint pains come and go suddenly.

Bryonia 30c: Intense fever, frontal or back headache, acute stitching pains, rapid, violent heartbeat; sour sweat worse from slightest motion even of breath.

Calc Carb 30c: Brought on maybe by working in water. Heat and sweat of head; cold, clammy feet and hands; violent perspirations about 3 A.M. Pain is worse from movement.

Rhus Tox 30c: Relief from continued motion; worse damp weather, cold, and approaching storm. Tearing pains with paralyzed sensation and stitches. (Follows Bryonia well.)

Streptococcin 200c: For complications or lack of recuperation (for 200c potency, see page 13).

(Other useful remedies: Arnica, Colchicum, Dulcamara, Pulsatilla, Sulphur, Spigelia.)

CELL SALTS

Ferr Phos: For first stage of fever, congestion and pain; rapid, throbbing pulse. Alternate Ferr Phos with Kali Mur when above fever signs occur with inflamed joints and swelling. Thumping pulse heard all over body. Thickening of tissues during fever.

Calc Phos: Weight loss, debility, rundown, and exhausted. When fever comes on very slowly alternate Calc Phos with Nat Phos.

Nat Phos: Sour-smelling sweat; creamy-yellow tongue; acid taste in mouth.

Ringworm

Caused by a fungus often transferred from a young animal.

DESCRIPTION

Small, circular patches of raised skin—rose-colored and scaly. The centers heal, leaving red rings. On the scalp it appears as small, round, bald patches. Usually appears first on head (in hair), then on chest, back of abdomen, and often the groin. However, any area can become affected. It is contagious on contact.

WHAT TO DO—INTERNAL APPLICATION

- Wash the infected part every day with soap and water. Use separate towels, washcloths, etc.
- Keep the area dry and exposed to air or sunlight.
- Change clothing (especially socks) frequently and whenever sweaty.
- Check animals to prevent cross-infection.

HERBS

Antiseptic: Golden Seal. Use as a tea and also to rinse the infected scalp.

Blood purifier for ringworm: Poke Root

WHAT TO DO—EXTERNAL APPLICATION

Clean and dry affected skin with Thuja tincture. Oil of lavender, Teatree, or Thyme can be applied together or separately (2 drops of each to 3 tsp. Olive or Soya oil).

HOMEOPATHIC

Bacillinum 200c: For ringworm (for 200c Potency, see page 13).

Sepia 30c: For isolated ringworm-type spots. May be itching, redness, and rawness.

CELL SALTS

Take each of the following three times daily: Kali Mur, Kali Sulph, Nat Phos, and Silica.

Rubella

An infectious disease.

Rubella (German Measles) is an acute, infectious disease, milder but sometimes difficult to distinguish from measles (see also Scarlet Fever).

DESCRIPTION

Begins as a mild headache and fever (99.5–101°F), stiff neck, slightly runny nose, and dry throat. The glands are often swollen behind the ears.

A rash appears on the face and neck on the first day, then moves to the trunk and limbs. There may be fine, pink spots around the mouth and some pinkness of the eyes though not weeping.

The rash and fever seldom last more than five days. Rubella is more severe in females.

Most common season: spring or early summer.
Incubation period: 2–3 weeks.
Isolation period: until rash fades.
Recovery time: 2–5 days.

WHAT TO DO

HERBS

For fever: Catnip, Yarrow, Boneset, or Lemon Balm
To help relax: Elder or Chamomile
To relieve pain: Jamaica Dogwood or Hops
To provide extra nourishment during illness: Lavender, Thyme, or Juniper. Combine your choice of herbs and have child sip warm throughout the day. Sweeten with honey, if desired.

HOMEOPATHIC

After suspected contact, see Resistance and Immunity, page 19.
Rubella 200c (Nosode—see page 21.): To help clear a severe case or for lingering aftereffects of the disease. *Do not give while disease is incubating.*
For other useful remedies, see Measles.

CELL SALTS

Ferr Phos: Gradual onset, fever, rosy spots on cheeks, chilly with sweats, wants head cool.
Kali Mur: For coated tongue, swollen glands, and runny nose. Alternate with Ferr Phos if these symptoms exist.

Note: There is great danger of fetal deformity if pregnant women are exposed to Rubella, especially during the first trimester.

SEEK MEDICAL OR HOMEOPATHIC ASSISTANCE.

TO BUILD RESISTANCE

To help strengthen the immune system and restore to full health after the disease (or vaccination), see page 19.

S

Scabies

A skin infection by a parasite called an itch mite.

The female is just visible to the naked eye, yellowish-white with eight legs. She burrows into the skin and lays her eggs, then dies. The eggs hatch in six days and leave the burrow in larval form, growing quickly to adults so the disease may be fully developed in two weeks.

Spread by close bodily contact with an infected person and only seldom through infected bedding, etc.

Scratching can cause severe inflammation or secondary infection such as impetigo (school sores).

DESCRIPTION

Intense itching, especially when child is warm. The burrow in the skin is distinctive and seen as a grayish or white hairlike line, often zigzag, about 0.5–1 cm along the skin with a dark speck at the farthest end (the eggs). Usually found in webs and sides of fingers, backs of hands, lower abdomen, penis and lower buttocks, underarms, elbows, and on palms and soles in younger children.

WHAT TO DO

- Daily washing of body and clothes is essential.
- Keep clothes and bedding separate to prevent possible spreading.
- Lemon and Garlic juice mixed together makes a useful application to affected parts.

HERBS

Internally: Internal cleansers may help make conditions unpleasant in the skin layers and help drive the mites out. A mixture of Elecampane Root, Fumitory, Figwort, and Aniseed can be drunk as a tea daily.

Externally: Oils of Clove, Lavender, Thyme, and/or Peppermint (1–2 drops) mixed with Soya or Almond oil are rubbed into affected parts several times daily.

Tansy tincture or infusion can be added to bathwater or used to bathe body.

HOMEOPATHIC

Arsen Alb 30c: Eruption on bends of knees: pustular eruptions with burning and itching, worse from external warmth.

Lycopodium. 30c: Violent itching causing thickening of skin; worse from warmth of bed and hot applications; better when uncovered.

Mercurius 30c: Itching that is worse in bends of elbows; large, pustular eruptions.

Sulphur 30c: Tingling and itching with burning and soreness after scratching.

Psorinum 200c: For repeated outbreaks of single, pustular spots after main eruption has gone (for 200c potency, see page 13).

(Others: Nux Vornica, Hepar Sulph, Causticum.)

CELL SALTS

Calc Sulph taken internally 3–4 times daily; can also be crushed and applied locally to the affected parts.

NOTE: Hydrocortisone creams may be effective in the short term but can worsen the condition in the long run.

Scarlet Fever

An infectious disease.

An acute disease caused by a streptococcal bacteria producing a fever, sore throat, and characteristic rash.

DESCRIPTION

Begins abruptly with headache, vomiting, fiery-looking throat with gradually increasing severity. The tongue is furry, and throat and palate become bright red.

On the second day, the child has a bright, deeply flushed face ("scarlet face"), except an oval white area around their bright red lips. The rash is flushed skin with minute points of intense red that usually starts on the neck and spreads over the body and limbs. It does not occur on the palms and soles. After about a week, the rash fades from the neck and peeling begins and may continue for several weeks.

Most common season: winter (and maybe autumn).

Incubation period: 1–7 days.

Isolation period: For seven days from the date of onset of the disease and until all symptoms have subsided, all abnormal discharges have ceased, and all open lesions have healed.

Recovery time: About three weeks.

Complications: Rheumatic fever, nephritis, ear infection, sinusitis, pneumonia.

WHAT TO DO

SEEK MEDICAL ADVICE IMMEDIATELY.

The following procedures can be helpful in restoring to full health *after medical treatment* or *until medical aid arrives*.

Restricted diet during high fever: fresh fruit, vegetables, soups, and freshly squeezed fruit or vegetable juices, or water. By taking no proteins, the body can use its energy to fight off the infection instead of digesting unnecessary food.

HERBS

To cleanse: Golden Seal, Dock, Mullein, and/or Red Clover
To provide extra nourishment: Lavender, Juniper, and/or Thyme
To soothe: Slippery Elm or Marshmallow

HOMEOPATHIC

After suspected contact, see Resistance and Immunity, page 19.

Apis 30c: High fever, no thirst, prickly skin, scanty urine; child is drowsy, restless, and agitated.
Belladonna 30c: Sore throat, strawberry tongue, swollen glands; rash is smooth and bright red. Delirium.
Bryonia 30c: For very slow appearance of rash; or sudden disappearance of rash with onset of complications.
Chamomilla 30c: If throat becomes ulcerated and child has a suffocative cough.
Rhus Tox 30c: Child is drowsy, weak, depressed, and restless; tongue is red and smooth, eruption does not appear.
Sulphur 30c: If rash is rough and dark-colored.
Scarletinum 200c (Nosode—see page 21): To help clear a severe case or for lingering aftereffects of the disease. Do *not give while disease is incubating.*

CELL SALTS

Ferr Phos: High temperature, headache, sore throat.
Kali Mur and Kali Sulph: Alternate every two hours after Ferr Phos.
Calc Phos: For convalescence period.
Kali Phos: If exhaustion is extreme, with putrid sore throat— give half-hourly until improvement.

HEALING YOUR CHILD

SEEK MEDICAL ADVICE IMMEDIATELY.

Symptoms of swollen neck glands, earache, dark-red or smoky urine, swelling around eyes or painful joints can indicate complications such as rheumatic fever, nephritis, ear infection, sinusitis, pneumonia.

TO BUILD RESISTANCE

To strengthen the immune system and help restore to full health after the disease, see page 19.

Shock

A condition caused by a lack of blood supply resulting in a lowering of the activities of the vital functions. It may be the result of illness, stress, injury, bleeding, burns, repeated vomiting, diarrhea, severe pain, heart failure, or allergic reactions (e.g., to bee stings).

DESCRIPTION

- Skin is pale, cold and clammy, with profuse sweating.
- May feel faint or giddy or have blurred vision.
- May feel sick and vomit.
- May be thirsty.
- May be anxious.
- Pulse tends to increase in rate but weaken as shock deepens.
- Breathing is shallow and rapid.

WHAT TO DO

1. *Seek expert help.*
2. Lay patient down in Recovery Position, with head lower than rest of the body and turned to the side if possible with one leg tucked up (unless unconscious, vomiting, or if injuries

make this inappropriate).

3. Reassure and give Aconite 200c (for 200c Potency, see page 13).
4. Loosen clothing at the neck, chest, and waist.
5. If thirsty, moisten lips with water.
6. Protect with blanket or sheet where needed.
7. Keep record of pulse and breathing rates.

HOMEOPATHIC

Aconite 30c: Shock with great fearfulness and anxiety.
Arnica 200c: If as the result of any injury.
Carbo Veg 30c: Extreme cases, semiconscious; cold breath and body; pale or blue.
Coca 30c: Altitude sickness, confusion, double vision.
Ignatia 30c: Emotional shock.
Veratrum Album 30c: Restless, chilly, profuse cold sweat, watery diarrhea.

See: **Emergency use of Homeophathy, p. 114.**

Sinusitis

An inflammatory condition of the sinuses occurring during common colds and nasal catarrh. Due to a streptococcal, staphylococcal, or pneumococcal infection.

DESCRIPTION

Starts as a heavy feeling in the face and head, especially when bending forward. First, a copious discharge from the nose. Next, the nasal passages swell and mucous or pus collect in the sinus cavities behind the nose and cause great distress. The resultant pressure causes severe tenderness, pain, and headache, sometimes toothache. Whereas a cold should clear up in a few days, untreated sinusitis can last for weeks.

WHAT TO DO

- Exercise, good ventilation, nourishing diet.
- Avoid mucous-forming foods, especially dairy foods.
- Drainage points on the face can provide relief when massaged. Massage drainage points by applying on/off pressure (3–second intervals) down sides of nose, along cheekbones, around bony orbits of eyes and temples as often as needed for relief.

HERBS

As antiseptic and to help fight infection: Echinacea, Garlic

If eyes are affected: Eyebright
To clear overloaded lymphatic system: Poke Root
To help dry out tissues and remove catarrh: Golden Seal, Bayberry, Elder, Golden Rod, Yarrow
To soothe inflamed surfaces: Marshmallow

Inhalation: Peppermint, Eucalyptus, and/or Teatree oils (4 drops) can be added to a bowl of steaming water and breathed in while holding towel over head to retain steam.

Externally: Rub above-mentioned oils on painful parts (1 drop of each to 2 Tbs. Soya or Almond oil).

HOMEOPATHY

Hepar Sulph 30c: Pain in facial bones; boring pain in upper lids worse from dry, cold winds and drafts. Red, inflamed eyes and lids; sore nostrils with thick discharge.
Iodum 30c: Sneezing; dry nose, fluent and hot in the open air; helps relieve a copious discharge; pain in eyes; throbbing head as of tight band; pain at root of nose and frontal sinuses; loss of smell.
Kali Bich 30c: Pressure and pain at root of nose. Thick greenish-yellow discharge. Sore nasal bones; tough elastic plugs leaving raw surface. Violent sneezing. Profuse, watery or

stopped-up sensation. Headache over eyebrows with aching and fullness worse over left eye.

Kali Iod 30c: Violent headache; pain through sides of head over eyes and root of nose; red, swollen nose. Profuse, hot, watery discharge. Sneezing, stuffy, or dry with no discharge.

Nat Mur 30c: Tears stream down face. Violent, fluent discharge, thin and watery like raw egg white; loss of smell and taste.

Phosphorus 30c: Oversensitive smell; chronic catarrh; tired eyes worse from light; fullness in head.

CELL SALTS

Ferr Phos: Fever and congestion; pain in sinuses; flushed face; rapid pulse; throbbing pain.

Kali Mur: Dull pain in sinus; thick, white discharge; stuffed-up head.

Nat Mur: Nasal obstruction, loss of smell; sensation of beating hammers in nose, worse from cold air.

Kali Sulph: Yellow, slimy discharge, worse in warm room and evening.

Silica: Chronic thick, offensive, acrid discharge; ulceration of mucous membranes; chronic nasal catarrh.

SEEK HOMEOPATHIC OR MEDICAL ADVICE if condition fails to respond in a week.

Sleep

1 Insomnia
2 Nightmares

1 Insomnia

Children who are happy and active during the day are probably getting enough sleep. Children have differing sleep requirements, with some children needing a lot less sleep than others of the same age and size.

Sleep provides rest for the brain and nervous system.

Insomnia is caused by a functional disturbance of the brain— the bloodflow to the brain doesn't slow down as it should at bedtime.

Possible causes: Putting children to bed before they are tired; physical discomfort; excess noise; extreme temperatures; hunger; digestive disturbances; fear; worry; overexcitement (e.g., after stimulating games or television programs); inability to relax.

WHAT TO DO

- Prolonged use of sedatives may be harmful and addictive.
- A warm bath with 2–3 drops of Lavender oil or Valerian tea added to bathwater.
- Cool bath and brisk skin rub in the morning. Adequate ventilation in the bedroom.
- A light evening meal (preferably no more than two hours before bedtime).
- If child has no allergy problems, a hot milk drink can be relaxing.
- Adequate exercise during the day but not overstimulation, as overtiredness can also contribute to insomnia.
- Reading a bedtime story initiates a "slowing down" process and gives the child quality time with the parent.

HERBS

The following Calcium-rich herbs help calm the nervous system: Valerian, Hops, Catnip, Chamomile, and/or Passionflower may be taken in the evening before bedtime.

HOMEOPATHIC

Aconite 30c: Restless sleep, tossing and turning, worse from fear or fright.

Arsen Alb 30c: Very anxious and restless, cannot stand to lie in bed, worse after midnight.

Coffea 30c: Cannot rest the mind, worse from excitement. Acute senses, hears distant noises distinctly.

Ignatia 30c: Worse from grief, e.g., during parents' absence.

Nux Vomica 30c: Cross and tired in the morning. May waken with headache. Sleepy in the early evening but wakens 3–4 A.M.

Pulsatilla 30c: Wide awake in the early evening before midnight.

Sulphur 30c: Catnaps; slightest noise awakens, then going back to sleep is very difficult.

CELL SALTS

Ferr Phos: Drowsy in the daytime, but sleepless at night.

Kali Phos: For children who cry and scream during sleep; dream; twitch muscles; yawn; stretch or sleepwalk. Give with warm drink before bed and again in bed if necessary.

Nat Phos: Insomnia associated with stomach pain or discomfort.

Silica: For nervous excitable children who feel the cold.

2 Nightmares

- Child may wake crying or screaming from a bad dream.
- Child may scream, toss and turn, sit up and talk, but doesn't wake up or remember in the morning.
- Sleepwalking. Some causes: Excessive or unwise eating before bed; fever; fear of the dark; family stresses.

WHAT TO DO

HERBS

Take Vitamin B and C-rich herbs such as Mistletoe, Chamomile, Thyme, Valerian, Hops, or Skullcap (especially for sleepwalking).

HOMEOPATHIC

Calc Carb 30c: Horrid visions on opening eyes; jerks and jumps at noises; sleep talking, night sweats; confused and frightened on awakening.

Helleborus 30c: Uneasy sleep with dark floating visions; sudden screams but cannot be fully aroused.

Lycopodium 30c: Many frightful, anxious, vivid dreams of murder and accidents.

Phosphorus 30c: Constant dreams, irrational talking; starts up suddenly when falling asleep; anxious upon awakening.

Pulsatilla 30c: Jerking limbs, confused dreams; suddenly sitting up in sleep; maybe screaming during sleep.

Stramonium 30c: Half-slumber; intense fear of the dark and of shining objects; awakens terrified; dreams and visions when half asleep.

CELL SALTS

Calc Phos: Vivid dreams—dreams of fire and danger.

Kali Phos: Useful for sleepwalkers; highly-strung nervous children.

Nat Sulph: Heavy sleep with anxious and plentiful dreams.

Bach Flowers may also be useful to work on emotional aspects (books on Bach Flowers and the Bach Flower Remedies can be found in most health shops).

Spots and Rashes

This section gives possible causes for spots and rashes. Refer to individual headings elsewhere in the book for what to do.

ALLERGY

If none of the other possibilities prove to be the cause, or if rash appears only at certain seasons or after exposure to certain foods, suspect an allergy. See section on Allergy.

BITES

Usually obvious, as there are only a few in isolated areas.

CHICKEN POX

Small, raised, irritating spots that turn to watery blisters and form crusts. Usually start on the trunk, then the limbs and face. Can turn septic.

CONTACT DERMATITIS

May appear as any one of a range of pimples or rashes, and cause mild or severe irritation. Caused by sensitivity to a specific substance. To determine this, see section on Contact Dermatitis (page 236).

DIAPER RASH

Burnt skin on bottom and diaper area.

ECZEMA

Itchy, red skin that may weep a clear fluid after scratching; forms crusts when dry. Skin becomes less red, dry, and thickened. Starts in bends in knees and elbows in toddlers; cheeks and foreheads in babies.

HIVES

Very itchy red spots of varying sizes; may cover large parts of the body; they become swollen and elevated then disappear and reappear.

IMPETIGO

Red spots progress to watery blisters then pus-filled sores that discharge and spread the infection. This leaves raw skin, which eventually forms crusts. Usually starts around mouth and nose or in armpit and groin in babies.

MEASLES

Rash of red-pink blotches beginning on face or behind ears, maybe in the mouth and spreading to trunk and limbs. Accompanied by "cold" symptoms. High temperature; sore runny eyes irritated by sunlight. Rash becomes raised and blotchy.

PSORIASIS

Thick layer of silvery scales, mild itching if any; scratching easily causes bleeding; usually on knees, elbows, scalp, and trunk.

RINGWORM

A circular patch of raised, rose-colored, scaly skin. The center heals to form red, scaly rings. In the hair it leaves bald patches. Usually starts on head in hair, chest, back, and abdomen.

RUBELLA

Similar to measles, but with a milder illness; spots are smaller and a paler pink. Just before the rash appears, lymph nodes behind and below back of skull swell.

SCABIES

Distinguished by the burrow seen as a gray or white hairlike line along the skin about 0.5–1 cm long with a darker speck at the farthest end. Usually on any of the fingers, hands, underarms, elbows, soles of feet, and/or lower abdomen.

SCARLET FEVER

Small bright red spots that are close together, usually start on neck, back, and chest; accompanied by headache and vomiting, sore throat, high temperature; flushed skin but pallid around mouth.

Sprains and Strains

Sprain: Stretching or tearing of a ligament.
Strain: Overstretching of a muscle or tendon.
Causes: Both are caused by sudden wrenching or twisting of any joint.

DESCRIPTION

Pain, loss of power, tenderness. Worse when attempting to move the limb. With sprains there is marked swelling and discoloration due to bleeding beneath the surface.

WHAT TO DO

- If there is any external bleeding, deal with this first (see Wounds).
- Avoid massage.
- Apply the Accident Compensation Corporation's "RICE" Formula (the first five minutes is important):

  - Rest: Ensure that injured limb is completely rested.
  - Ice: Make an ice pack by crushing ice into towel or plastic bag, or by simply using a pack of frozen vegetables (oil can be put on to skin first, for sensitive skin).
  - Compression: Apply a pressure bandage around injury. Every four hours repeat ice packs followed by pressure bandage for first twenty-four hours.
  - Elevation: Keep the limb raised as much as possible.
- The healing process is greatly aided by stimulating the blood

204

flow and relaxing the tense muscles.

- After resting the injured limb twenty-four hours, continue the RICE treatment combined with *gentle* exercise. Take the limb through the normal range of movement, stop if pain is excessive, apply ice immediately after exercise.
- Do not force movement of the injured limb.

HERBS

To help reduce swelling and repair damaged tissue, apply a poultice of Chickweed, Comfrey, or Puriri.

If skin is not broken: Arnica ointment several times daily.

If skin is broken: Calendula ceam or lotion several times daily.

For pain: Oils of Wintergreen, Sage, Rosemary, or Thyme (5 drops mixed with 3 tsp. Olive or Soya oil) can be rubbed gently on to painful part. Avoid rubbing oil into deep cuts.

HOMEOPATHIC

Arnica 30c: For sudden wrenching of muscles with injuries to the soft tissues of the body. Half-hourly for 3–4 doses, followed by Rhus Tox 30c twice daily for 4–5 days.

Bryonia 30c: If swelling develops anywhere around injury site. After a few doses go back to Rhus Tox to help repair injury.

Ledum 30c: If affected parts feel numb or cold. Then resume taking Rhus Tox to help repair injury. Rhus Tox 30c: For injuries to ligaments and fibrous tissues.

Ruta Grav 30c: For old sprains causing lingering problems.

CELL SALTS

For Sprains:

Ferr Phos: Sprains, muscle pain, worse from movement.

Kali Mur: Sprains with bruising and swelling. These can be used internally and as a lotion to bathe the affected part (four crushed tablets mixed with half-cup of water).

For Strains Alternate Kali Mur and Calc Fluor for as long as needed.

SEEK MEDICAL ADVICE

- If there is no improvement after two days using above procedures.

T

Teeth

1 Teething
2 Toothache

1 Teething

There are a number of ways you can help your baby through the stressful and often painful periods of cutting teeth.

HERBS

Catnip or Chamomile tea is a safe and soothing drink for babies. This may be sweetened with honey, if desired. A few drops of Plantago tincture may be added to this drink, or rubbed onto the painful gum area to ease pain. Rub one drop of Clove oil on to gums.

HOMEOPATHIC

Calc Carb 30c: Difficult teething with lots of saliva and easy bleeding and swelling of gums, diarrhea. Stools sour with undigested food.

Calc Phos 30c: For slow teethers who are weak and tired during the teething stage. Foul, hot, spluttery stools may be watery. Teeth decay rapidly. These children are often slow in learning to walk.

Chamomilla 30c: One cheek may be red, hot, or swollen; child cries and is very dissatisfied; convulsions may accompany teething. Yellow-green slimy stools smelling like bad eggs. Pain is intolerable. Head and scalp are hot and sweaty.

Kreosotum 30c: Teeth decay rapidly; child worries and frets, must be patted all night.

CELL SALTS

Calc Phos: For slow cutting teeth; also for rapidly decaying teeth, or deformed teeth especially when accompanied by runny stools.

Calc Fluor: Vomiting and crying during teething. Lack of enamel.

Nat Mur: Constant dribbling of saliva during teething.

2 Toothache

Usually caused by decay. Take good care of first teeth. If they decay, then the second teeth will also be troublesome.

Toothache may also be caused by taking food or drink too hot or too cold, or exposure to cold air.

A decayed tooth must always be dealt with by a dentist or dental nurse.

WHAT TO DO

- Foods to ensure healthy teeth in the long term: almonds, apples, carrots, celery, cheese, buttermilk, nuts, oats, rye, radish, sunflower seeds, alfalfa.

HERBS

Combine your choice from the following lists:

For unhealthy, ulcerated, easy-bleeding gums, poor teeth and bad breath: Echinacea, Myrrh, or Poke Root

To ensure healthy teeth in the long term: Comfrey, Sage, Myrrh, Plantain and/or Yarrow

HEALING YOUR CHILD

To relieve acute pain: Lobelia, Clove, or Plantago tinctures—
1–2 drops on cotton applied directly to painful tooth

HOMEOPATHIC

Aconite 30c: For throbbing, burning pain.

Belladonna 30c: Throbbing gum, dry mouth, ulcerated gums.

Kreosotum 30c: Early decay of teeth; teeth turn yellow then dark.

Mercurius 30c: Aching teeth, worse at night with bad breath, moist mouth, easy bleeding and swelling of gums, inflamed or abscessed roots, increased salivation and sensation as if the teeth were too long or too loose.

Plantago 30c: Sensitive to touch, worse from cold air, better while eating.

Pulsatilla 30c: For unbearable pain, worse from heat, better from cold drink.

Silica 30c: Deep pain and ulceration of gums. Abscesses about roots of teeth.

CELL SALTS

Calc Phos: Useful after toothache to help purify blood throughout gums.

Calc Sulph: For abscessed gums that will not heal.

Kali Mur: Toothache with swollen gum or cheek.

Mag Phos: Nervous child with spasmodic, sharp, shooting pains. Better from hot applications.

Nat Mur: Toothache with excess saliva or tears, and easy-bleeding gums.

Silica: Deep-seated pain and ulcerated gums.

Pressure Point: Apply firm pressure to index finger on the lower corner of fingernail nearest the thumb; may be necessary to apply pressure to both hands.

Tetanus

A notifiable disease (must be reported to a medical doctor or local Health Department).

A neuromuscular disease caused by a bacteria that enters through slight cuts, ulcers, or burns, animal bites, or compound fractures. Smallpox vaccination can sometimes cause similar symptoms.

The tetanus organism is found everywhere, especially in manured soil, intestines of horses and cows, on unclean, unhealthy skin and in ear discharges of those with otitis media.

DESCRIPTION

Usually assumes three stages:

1. Back pain
2. Spasm of jaw and abdominal muscles, rigid movement
3. Convulsions

General symptoms are difficulty in opening mouth and swallowing (spasm of the jaw muscle); chills, pain in throat, backache, stiff neck, abdominal pain, fever, stiffness at site of injury, rigid facial and skeletal muscles.

Incubation period: From four days to four weeks. (A long incubation period has more favorable results.)
Recovery time: Five days to three weeks.
Complications: Respiratory, circulatory failure; urine retention, miscarriage in pregnancy, pneumonia.

WHAT TO DO

SEEK MEDICAL ADVICE IMMEDIATELY.
The following procedures can be helpful in restoring to full

health *after medical treatment or until medical aid arrives.*

HERBS

Lobelia tincture (1–2 drops) at half hourly intervals (some children react strongly to this herb, so it is wise to use a low dose).

To aid the nervous system: Yarrow, Valerian, Lavender and/or Marjoram

HOMEOPATHIC

After suspected contact, see Resistance and Immunity, page 19.

Aconite 30c: Sudden, violent invasion of symptoms: stiff neck, chilliness, abdominal colic; numb burning throat, with fever.

Cicuta 30c: If infected wound suddenly ceases to discharge, causing rigidity and distortion of limbs with staring eyes and difficult breathing.

Gelsemium 30c: For paralysis or spasm of muscles, difficult swallowing, chilliness, and trembling. Hypericum 30c: Wounds from sharp, dirty objects; shooting, violent, piercing pains. Also for jerking and lockjaw from injury to nerves, especially spinal nerves.

Ledum 30c: For deep puncture wounds, give 3 times daily for 3 days if tetanus is suspected, but before jerking symptoms appear.

Tetanotoxin 200c: (Nosode—see page 21): To help clear a severe case or for lingering aftereffects of the disease. *Do not give while disease incubating.*

CELL SALTS

Mag Phos: Give half-hourly at first sign of symptoms and until symptoms are cleared. This cell salt may also help reduce any ill effects from the vaccination.

TO BUILD RESISTANCE

To help strengthen the immune system and restore to full health after the disease (or vaccination), see page 19.

Throat (Sore)

May be the beginning of a cold or the first symptom of a more serious illness. Watch for changes in symptoms and check under Colds, Diphtheria, Scarlet Fever, Tonsillitis.

WHAT TO DO

- Gargle with 2 tsp. salt in 1 cup water: *do not swallow.*
- Gargle with 2 tsp. cider vinegar in 1 cup water.
- Drink hot lemon juice and honey.

HERBS

To soothe a sore throat: Hyssop, Coltsfoot, or Licorice.
To purify: Elecampane
To provide a natural source of vitamins and minerals: Sage and/or Thyme. These herbs work well when mixed, drunk hot, sweetened with honey.

Inhalation: Oils of Lemon, Sage, and/or Thyme (2 drops of each) added to a bowl of steaming water. Cover head with towel and breathe in the steam to loosen the congestion and ease the pain.

HOMEOPATHIC

To help prevent recurrent sore throats with constantly enlarged tonsils: Baryta Carb can be taken night and morning for three days, then once weekly during susceptible time of year.

Belladonna 30c: For throat that is sore, dry, red, and inflamed.

Causticum 30c: Raw and sore throat.

Hepar Sulph 30c: Sticking pain as of a splinter in throat.

Mercurius 30c: Red, swollen, painful, and very inflamed, with pains extending often to ears.

Rhus Tox 30c: Sore throat with swollen glands.

Streptococcin 30c: If throat has not been right since previous infection. Give once daily for two days. Repeat at a later date if necessary.

Tuberculinum 30c: Recurrent sore throat spreading to chest with rattling wheeze.

STREP THROAT

Begins with sudden sore throat and fever; often without the signs of a cold or cough. The back of the mouth and tonsils become very red, and the lymph glands under the jaw become swollen and tender. It is a potentially serious condition, different from sore throats.

WHAT TO DO

- If using homeopathic remedies, Streptococcin must be used in conjunction with the relevant remedy above.
- SEEK MEDICAL ATTENTION. If no improvement within twenty-four hours, the doctor will give child a throat swab and maybe penicillin. Untreated strep throat can be followed by rheumatic fever and glomerulonephritis 1–3 weeks later (these diseases cause heart valve problems and kidney failure).

Thrush

A fungal infection of the mucous membranes of the mouth in babies of both sexes or of vaginal tract in girls. The fungus is known as Candida Albicans.

DESCRIPTION

In mouth, thrush looks like milk curds, but these will not brush off and may bleed when rubbed. These white patches occur on tongue, gums, or throat. It may follow treatment by antibiotics. In vaginal infection, there is increased vaginal discharge and itching irritation outside the vagina.

WHAT TO DO

- If this fungus is not cleared adequately from the body, it can change into its mold form, which causes more deep-set problems including vitamin/mineral deficiencies and allergic reactions.
- Hygiene is important. Be sure to change underwear regularly.
- Natural yogurt can be very soothing when applied locally, but will not clear an established infection. Acidophyllus powder (break open a capsule) can be mixed with yogurt prior to application for better results.
- Calendula or Hypericum creams can be soothing when applied locally.

HERBS

Herbs to be used as a mouthwash, and/or drink:

Antiseptic: Golden Seal and/or Echinacea
To rinse mouth or vaginal area: oils of Lemon, Geranium, or
    Sage (5 drops to half-cup water).
To soothe irritation: Raspberry

HOMEOPATHIC

Candida Albicans 30c: Four times daily for two or three days. The liquid form of this remedy is better in this case, as the child with Candida overgrowth may not respond favorably to lactose (the base of homeopathic tablets).

Other useful remedies:

Arsen Alb 30c: Child thirsty for small amounts of water; great burning of affected parts.

Bryonia 30c: Nursing aggravates the sore mouth in babies.

Calc Carb 30c: For vaginal itching and whitish discharge.

Mercurius 30c: Gums are spongy, swollen, and the sores tend to ulcerate. Diarrhea may occur simultaneously.

To rinse mouth or vaginal area: Hypercal lotion can be diluted (5 drops to half-cup water).

CELL SALTS

Kali Mur: Will help soothe the itch. Suck tablets and use as wash (crush four tablets to half-cup water).

Seek Further Advice

- For stubborn recurring cases.
- There are advanced balancing techniques now available that enable the body to repel the invasion of Candida Albicans.

Tonsillitis

A specific infection of the tonsillar tissues (these are two small lumps visible on each side of the throat near the base of the tongue) and associated glands.

Usually a streptococcal infection that some children cannot easily fight off.

DESCRIPTION

Acute Tonsillitis: Fever, loss of appetite, coated tongue, difficulty swallowing, maybe headache and vomiting. When pushing down on the tongue with a spoon handle, the sidewalls of the throat appear red, swollen, possibly with whitish-yellow spots. In younger children, there may also be abdominal pains.

Chronic Tonsillitis: Less severe than acute condition but more persistent. General ill health, easily tired, poor appetite, repeated sore throats, low-grade fever, and enlarged neck glands. Adenoids often enlarge with chronic tonsillitis, which can cause blockage of air through the nose. This results in mouth breathing, producing a nasal voice and snoring. Repeated ear infections are more common.

Complications: Ear infections, rheumatic fever, and inflammation of the kidneys.

WHAT TO DO

- For chronic tonsillitis, we advise that you seek the help of an experienced natural health practitioner.
- Give child mainly liquid foods such as fresh, unsweetened juices and soups, plus fresh fruit and vegetables until acute symptoms subside.
- Best foods are carrot, celery, beetroot, pineapple, lemon, and coconut milk. Hot lemon and honey drinks.
- Cider vinegar gargle to break up mucous (1 tsp. per half-cup water).
- Cool compress to throat at night, if throat feels hot, or child desires it.

HERBS

Antiseptics, blood purifiers, and soothing herbs are best suited. In chronic cases, continue for three weeks, stop one week, and repeat again.

Make a mixture of any of the following blood-purifying herbs: Golden Seal, Burdock, Echinacea, Poke Root, Queens Delight (especially if ears are involved).

To help soothe inflamed surfaces: Marshmallow, Licorice,

and/or Slippery Elm.

To provide extra nourishment: Rosemary, Cloves, and/or Teatree.

HOMEOPATHIC

Arsen Alb 30c: Burning, swollen throat better from warmth; worse from cold and swallowing.

Baryta Carb 30c: Constantly enlarged tonsils. Also glands of neck and behind ear are swollen. Helps remove a predisposition to tonsillitis.

Belladonna 30c: Dry and angry looking but inclined to swallow often, sharp pains in tonsils.

Hepar Sulph 30c: Sensation of splinter in throat, or sharp, throbbing pains with formation of pus.

Lachesis 30c: Bluish-red swelling, worse from anything tight around throat, worse from hot drinks or swallowing, and worse in the morning.

Mercurius 30c: Raw, burning, maybe yellow spots, stitching feeling toward ear on swallowing. Enlarged tonsils may cause difficulty in breathing.

Rhus Tox 30c: For chronic tendency to sore throat with loss of appetite.

Streptococcin 200c: For lack of reaction or if there is a history of streptococcal infections (for 200c potency see page 13).

CELL SALTS

Ferr Phos: For first signs of throat problem, take internally and use as a gargle (four tablets crushed and mixed with half-cup water).

Calc Phos: If swelling has continued for a long time.

Calc Sulph: If pus forms.

Kali Mur: Swollen tonsils, painful swallowing, white tongue.

Nat Phos: Yellow coating at base of tongue, with feeling of lump in throat.

- For developing earache or rash, marked swelling of neck glands, swollen joints, dark red or smoky urine passed in small amounts.

See also: Strep Throat, page 213.

Travel Sickness

The rhythmic or irregular movement associated with traveling affects the balance mechanism of the inner ear and, via the nerves, disturbs the digestive system, causing nausea and vomiting.

WHAT TO DO

- Plenty of fresh air in the vehicle.
- Keep mind busy and stretch legs to keep up circulation; reading tends to make the problem worse.
- Have child exert on/off pressure firmly at the following places: Find the little dent on the skull about half an inch back from the ear; also press with fingertips firmly into the middle of the tummy just below the rib cage.
- Special strips available from pharmacists give relief when placed on wrists. These work on the principle of acupuncture.

HERBS

- Have child sip tea made from Clove, Peppermint, Basil, and Cinnamon half an hour before traveling.
- Combine or use separately, and place 3–4 drops on handkerchief to sniff during the journey: Clove, Peppermint, Basil, and Cinnamon oils.

HOMEOPATHIC

Give the remedy you choose, once the night before and once on the morning of the journey; also once when the journey begins. If the journey is long, you may need to repeat the dose at half-hour intervals.

Belladonna 30c: Air sickness or earache from pressure during flying.

Borax 30c: Worse from downward motion in cars or planes.

Cocculus 30c: Worse from food smells and watching motion; nausea with faintness, vomiting and trembling; better lying down.

Ipecac 30c: Heavy vomiting associated with travel sickness.

Petroleum 30c: Empty feeling, nausea with empty stomach; worse from fumes, light, noise, and sitting up.

Tabacum 30c: Seasickness; icy, cold sweat; nausea; terrible, faint, sick feeling at pit of stomach; worse having eyes open and better from fresh air.

CELL SALTS

Nat Phos and Kali Phos together at half-hourly intervals. Give these half an hour before leaving also.

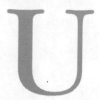

Urinary Tract Infection (Cystitis)

The urinary tract can cope with a few germs, but if the body defenses are down and excess germs build up in the urethra, an infection can get underway. As the infection spreads, the bladder loses its ability to hold increasing amounts of urine without discomfort. Urination becomes painful and is followed by painful spasms. Infection can eventually travel to kidney, causing back pain, elevated temperature, sweating, shivering, headaches, and general ill feeling.

WHAT TO DO—INTERNAL APPLICATION

- *Drink a little water often.*
- Acidify the urine by drinking 2 tsp. Apple Cider vinegar with 1 tsp. natural honey in a glass of water with each meal.
- Keep genital area clean, especially in girls; wash well; wipe from front to back after bowel movements, *not* back to front.

HERBS

It is advisable to continue taking the herbs for several weeks.

For infection: Uva Ursi and Buchu
To help cleanse and ease the passage of urine: Lavender and/or Juniper
To soothe the irritated area: Marshmallow

WHAT TO DO—EXTERNAL APPLICATION

Oils of Lavender or Juniper (2 drops) can be mixed with 3 tsp. Olive or Soya oil and rubbed on to the lower abdomen often.

Chronic Cystitis

When the above herbs fail to be of any use, change to regular drinks of Echinacea, Burdock, Golden Seal, and Myrrh. These act as a natural antibiotic.

HOMEOPATHIC

Aconite 30c: Burning, cutting, scanty urine with agony beforehand.

Belladonna 30c: Cramps in bladder with frequent, profuse, dark urine. Sensation of something moving inside.

Berberis 30c: If the pains have moved to the back or hips as well as the bladder region. Sticking, tearing pain worse from deep pressure. Cutting pain in bladder with burning on urinating. Back feels stiff and numb.

Cantharis 30c: Violent inflammation with intolerable urging. May be blood in the urine. Urine is passed in drops, with intense burning on urinating. Aching in small of back.

Staphysagria 30c: For sexually active teenagers whose symptoms are those from sexual activity.

Tuberculinum 200c: Chronically recurring cystitis, when above remedies fail (for 200c potency, see page 13). Then go back to the indicated remedy if infection recurs.

CELL SALTS

Kali Phos: Itching, scalding, bloody urine, cutting pain.

Mag Phos: Painful straining, severe spasms.

Nat Mur: Frequent with burning, cutting pain.

SEEK ADVICE

- Consult a doctor if child has bloody urine.
- For recurrent infections, your local medical doctor will take a urine culture before advising; a homeopath may also be able to help remove the cause of the problem.

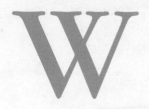

Warts

A common viral disease of the skin. Left untreated, warts may spontaneously remit in about eighteen months because the body develops an immunity to the wart virus. Few warts are contagious.

WHAT TO DO

Vitamin E capsules can be squeezed on and covered with a plaster. Repeat continuously for 2–3 weeks. Aloe Vera can be applied the same way.

HERBS

- Greater Celandine leaves can be picked and the yellow sap squeezed on to the wart daily until wart goes.
- Thuja tincture can be painted directly on to warts.
- The juice of the Milkweed can be applied directly to warts daily.
- Lemon oil can be dabbed on before bed every night.

HOMEOPATHIC

Causticum 30c: Small warts all over the body, especially nose, fingertips, eyebrows.
Ferr Pic 30c: Warts cover the hands.
Nat Mur 30c: For warts on the palms.
Nitric Acid 30c: Large, jagged, easy-bleeding warts.
Thuja 30c: A general wart treatment. Warts can be large and painful.

CELL SALTS

Kali Mur and Silica: One tablet of each three times daily.

NOTE: "Magic" cures are many, varied, and at times successful, and should not be discounted.

Whooping Cough

An infectious disease.

An acute, infectious disease affecting the air passages with characteristic coughing spasms.

DESCRIPTION

Appearing in stages:

Stage 1: This stage lasts from 3–7 days and consists of a runny nose, sneezing, slight fever, and cough that is worse at night, comes in spasms, and becomes progressively stronger.

Stage 2: During the second week, the coughs are so close together that the child cannot draw another breath and appears to be suffocating. The air is then sucked in with such force that it produces the characteristic whoop. After several such spasms (lasting 2–3 minutes) the child perspires, brings up some thick, slimy mucous, and may vomit food. This leaves the child exhausted and frightened but he/she recovers and can be quite happy between attacks. There may be 40–50 attacks daily.

Young infants and immunized children who develop whooping cough may have all the symptoms without the whoop.

Most common season: spring and autumn.
Age: under five.
Incubation period: 7–14 days.
Isolation period: for three weeks from the date of onset of the typical spasms.

Recovery time: mild cases with no whoop, 7–10 days. More serious cases can last from three weeks to two months.

Complications: Pneumonia, convulsions, and measles—all of which, in combination with whooping cough, are very serious; also dehydration, malnutrition, and bloody nose.

WHAT TO DO

- Give fluids—fresh fruit and vegetable juices, broths. Overloading the stomach with food is to be avoided.
- Avoid cold drafts.
- Keep warm and well rested.
- Be prepared for vomiting.
- Reassure child during spasms: *support—do not suffocate.*

HERBS

Make a mixture from the following:

To calm the child: Chamomile or Lavender
To purify glands: Red Clover or Thyme
To soothe respiratory passages: Mullein or Marshmallow
To tonify the system: Gentian

HOMEOPATHIC

After suspected contact, see Resistance and Immunity, page 19.

Antim Tart 30c: Worse from drinking and eating, cries before cough, vomits large amounts of mucous; nausea and cold sweat, white-coated tongue.

Belladonna 30c: Stomach pain and tears before spasm, dry throat, coughs until mucous comes up, excited by tickling in throat.

Bryonia 30c: Must sit up to cough. Coughing and vomiting occurs during a meal, yet child can return easily to finish the meal.

Carbo Veg 30c: When child is absolutely worn out, pale, and exhausted from the disease.

Cuprum 30c: For convulsions following a coughing spasm.

Drosera 30c: Barking cough so frequent that child chokes; raising of phlegm ends in retching and vomiting, worse after midnight.

Ipecac 30c: Stiff and blue during spasms, with difficult breathing; nausea better from vomiting; copious discharge and perspiration; exhausted after attack.

Pertussin 200c (Nosode—see page 21): To help clear severe case or for lingering aftereffects of the disease. *Do not give while disease is incubating.* There are several whooping-cough-type viruses. Pertussin may not be the most appropriate remedy, so seek the guidance of a skilled homeopath.

CELL SALTS

Calc Phos: Weak constitution or lingering cases.

Kali Mur: Alternate with Mag Phos where there is thick, white mucous.

Mag Phos: For first sign of illness.

SEEK MEDICAL ADVICE IF

- Child has convulsions;
- Shortness of breath *between* spasms;
- The child becomes debilitated during the long illness.

TO BUILD RESISTANCE

To strengthen the immune system and restore to full health after the disease or vaccination, see page 19.

Worms

The most common worms are threadworms (6–9 mm long). These look like fine cotton threads. Eggs are laid on the outside of the anus and are transferred from there back to the mouth or to toys, etc.

DESCRIPTION

Itching around the anus, which may disturb the child's sleep. Child may grind teeth in sleep. Sometimes the worms move into the vagina, causing itching and discharge.

Examination of the stool will usually show fine moving threads; worms can often be seen around the anus while child is sleeping.

Symptoms are general irritability, usually large appetite with low corresponding weight gain; child bores fingers into nose; there may be dark rings under eyes.

WHAT TO DO

- Ensure the child washes hands with soap after going to the toilet.
- Keep fingernails short.
- Prevent the child from scratching; have them wear gloves if necessary.

HERBS

- Choose Wormwood, Tansy, and/or Southernwood and mix with Chamomile to improve the taste. Mix with honey if necessary and have child drink this 2–3 times daily until symptoms are clear.
- Further helpful herbs to be added and continued daily: Peppermint, Thyme, or Garlic.
- Raisins soaked in Senna tea may be an easy food for the young child.

Abrotanum 30c: Pale and old-looking face with blue rings around eyes; child is cross and peevish; ravenous hunger but no weight gain.

Absinthium 30c: Grinding teeth, loathing of food with uncomfortable, irritable feeling in stomach, and colic in abdomen.

Calc Carb 30c: Swollen abdomen; dark rings under deep-seated eyes; sore nostrils; ravenous hunger.

Cina 30c: Rings around eyes, grinds teeth; picks and rubs nose; night terrors; hungry soon after eating; itchy anus.

CELL SALTS

Kali Mur: Alternate with Nat Phos when child has an itching anus and white tongue.

Nat Phos: For round, long or thread worms, with squinting and twitching of facial muscles.

Give one tablet twice daily between meals. Stop and if no improvement after five days combine Nat Mur and Silica and take in the same dosage.

Wounds

1 Superficial (cuts and abrasions)
2 Deep (lacerations, incisions, punctures, contusions— internal hemorrhage)

1 Superficial Wounds

Where only the upper layers of the skin are damaged or removed; some bleeding occurs but mostly a clear fluid exudes. This may be from graze, or a slight cut with a sharp instrument.

• Clean using Hypercal lotion (10 drops to half-glass water) as antiseptic and healer, and follow if necessary with Calendula cream and plaster.

2 Deep wounds

Lacerations:

Full thickness of skin is cut through, often in an irregular fashion. Caused by a jagged or blunt instrument—infection is common. The edges can be pulled apart. There may be damage to the underlying tissues (muscles, nerves, blood vessels); these are often messy and contain dirt.

Incised wounds:

Skin is cut by a sharp instrument so that skin is divided and there may be damage to deeper tissues such as nerves, tendons, or blood vessels.

Punctures:

Skin is pierced by a sharp point such as a nail or rose thorn. There is damage to deep tissue and, as oxygen cannot get to the injured part, infection often results. This type of wound is particularly prone to the tetanus bacteria.

Contused wounds:

Internal hemorrhage—damage to the soft tissue beneath the skin. Caused by a knock from a blunt object. May be a cut but the more serious damage is beneath the skin, with pain, swelling, bruising, and thickening of tissues.

GENERAL PROCEDURE FOR ALL DEEP WOUNDS

1. SEEK MEDICAL ADVICE. Give Arnica 200c for shock and bleeding (for 200c potency, see page 13).
2. CONTROL BLEEDING

    - *Elevate the part* with cut surface uppermost.
    - *If blood is bright red,* it is from an artery. Ensure there is nothing sharp in the wound, carefully remove any

foreign objects that can be *easily* picked out, then apply pressure around wound.

- *If blood is dark,* it is from a vein and only light pressure is necessary.
- *If you suspect a fracture or if a bone or sharp object is poking through,* apply pressure alongside object or bone, place pads of cotton or soft material round the wound to a height to prevent pressure on object or bone; bandage diagonally so as to slow bleeding but not press on object.
- Bleeding can be stopped by applying pressure at an appropriate point between heart and wound. Do not apply pressure for more than fifteen minutes.
- *For contused wounds,* elevate the part and apply ice packs (or ice in plastic bag) and a firm bandage.

3. CLEAN THE WOUND when bleeding has stopped, with cotton soaked in one of the following:

- Hypercal lotion (5 drops in half-glass water)
- Comfrey lotion (see Herbs page 8)
- Teatree oil (3 drops to half-cup water)

Gently stroke foreign matter out, using a clean cotton ball for each stroke.

NOTE: Do not use Arnica on an open wound. If child's cuts tend to go septic, place a few drops of Urtica Urens or Hypercal lotion in the daily bathwater.

Compress or ointment

To disinfect and prevent infection: Golden Seal, Elecampane, Sage, or Lavender

To help heal: Calendula, Comfrey

To soothe the wound: Marshmallow, Comfrey, or Slippery Elm

4. BANDAGING. Soak a piece of gauze or lint in lotion made from your chosen herbs. Cover entire wound. Repeat with a

second piece of gauze (this can be replaced later without disturbing the dressing immediately next to the skin). Bandage firmly or use butterfly bandages. (These can be easily made by cutting bandage into butterfly shape.)

5. IF WOUND BECOMES INFLAMED, i.e., red and hot with swelling and tenderness, or starts discharging, remove outer gauze and replace with clean gauze soaked in Hypercal lotion or above-mentioned herbs. Rebandage. Give homeopathic Hepar Sulph 30c three times daily until discharge stops. However, if no improvement after two or three days, treat for infection.

6. WHEN WOUND BEGINS TO HEAL, it can gradually be exposed to the air, as oxygen plays an important part in the healing process.

INTERNAL APPROACH TO HELP HEAL WOUNDS

HERBS

Comfrey, Elecampane, Golden Seal, and Rosemary can be taken as a tea to help fight infection from within.

HOMEOPATHIC

Lacerations
Often require skilled surgical treatment.

Arnica 200c: For shock and to help control bleeding (for 200c potency, see page 13).
Hypericum 30c: If pain is severe.

Incised Wounds
Staphysagria 30c: For very deep painful wounds.

Puncture Wounds
Ledum 30c: To help guard against any tetanus bacteria. Four times daily for two days.
Hypericum 30c: Use instead of Ledum especially for shooting

pains in the wound. This will also help guard against tetanus bacteria.

Contused Wounds/Internal Hemorrhage

Arnica 200c three times in one day followed by Arnica 30c for the next few days to allay pain and promote absorption of blood.

Give Ledum 30c if parts feel numb and cold and if there is delay in appearance of the bruise. Apply Arnica ointment externally also if the skin is not broken.

Veratrum Album 30c: Internal bruising where swelling and pain occurs.

Blows to Chest

Bryonia 30c

Blows to Head

Nat Sulph 30c

Blows to Abdomen

Veratrum Album 30c

CELL SALTS

Calc Sulph: For those wounds that are filled with pus.

Ferr Phos: For first stage of cuts, bruises, falls, and sprains.

Kali Mur: Give for swellings.

Alternate Kali Phos and Nat Phos for signs of infection (e.g., redness and swelling).

Silica: For neglected wounds that are slow to heal, or infected.

SEEK MEDICAL ADVICE.

- If you suspect damage to deeper structures, or internal hemorrhage. Symptoms of this will be pain, tenderness, cold clammy skin; restlessness; thirst; or dizziness and fainting.

- If despite above procedures, there is increased pulse; paleness; distressed breathing or a deteriorating condition.
- If foreign body is embedded—this may be large or small (e.g., pieces of glass).

Miscellaneous
Ailments

Bad Breath

This can be seen as an early warning sign and may indicate liver trouble, inadequate digestion of food, tooth decay, respiratory problems, gum infection, inflammation of the throat, catarrhal discharge, or sinus trouble. It is wise to seek advice from a natural health practitioner at this early stage to help isolate the cause.

Contact Dermatitis

Inflammation of the skin, arising from touching a substance to which the person is sensitive. The eruption appears within a few minutes to hours after contact or application, developing rapidly and vanishing some variable time after removal of the cause.

DESCRIPTION

The eruption may be spotty, discolored, raised or flat, bleeding or pus filled, pimples, blisters, or cuts.

Sensations present upon the skin may be: itching, pricking, tingling, smarting, burning, pain. Variations in intensity of these sensations depend upon susceptibility and sensitivity of the individual.

WHAT TO DO

- A patch test, where the suspected substance is applied to scratched skin, will usually cause a reaction within twenty minutes (place on soft skin like wrist).
- Seek advice from a Touch for Health instructor. (Muscle testing will isolate suspect substances which then need to be eliminated or rebalanced.)

HOMEOPATHY

Homeopathy offers antidotes to the offending substances to counteract ill effects. And, even if the cause is eliminated, homeopathic remedies are often helpful in restoring the skin to normal by treating the whole constitution.

Herbal lotion to give relief in the meantime: 3 tsp. either of cold-pressed Soya, Almond, or Castor oil mixed with one drop each of oil of Lavender and Geranium.

Chamomile and Hyssop extracts are also soothing.

Growing Pains

Any unexplained, vague, temporary bone pains that the child complains of, providing such pains do not follow an acute illness (e.g., rheumatic fever) or an injury (e.g., broken bones), are usually called "growing pains" and can often be helped by:

- Daily drinks of Parsley tea which is rich in vitamins and minerals
- Calc Phos Cell salt taken three times daily
- Homeopathic Phosphoric Acid, Guiacum, Calc Phos 30c, or Belladonna 200c
- A few drops of Lavender or Thyme oil can be rubbed on to the affected area to soothe.

Seek medical or homeopathic advice if pains persist.

Head Lice

A form of louse (Pediculosis Capitis) that lives exclusively on the scalp. The adult lice are light green in color, visible to the naked eye, and live at the base of the hair. They lay their white eggs on the hair shaft and reproduce rapidly. They spread mostly through personal contact or by the use of infested head garments, combs, pillows, etc.

DESCRIPTION

The white, glistening nit or egg can be found glued firmly and in great numbers to the hair shaft, especially around the ears and in mid-back of head. Severe itching of scalp. Constant and vigorous scratching causes oozing of a fluid that is watery at first but in severe cases contains blood or pus. The fluid dries and forms crusts or may remain sticky and mat the hair.

WHAT TO DO

Most schoolchildren are regularly checked to guard against infestations. A medical shampoo can be obtained from pharmacies to kill the nits.

During treatment, keep bedding, brushes, combs, etc. clean and separate to avoid cross-infection.

HERBS

- Apply Aniseed oil to the infested areas to kill nits and eggs; or mix one part Sassafras tincture with two parts Olive oil and rub over scalp before shampooing, four times weekly. Comb with a fine-tooth comb to remove dead lice and eggs. Repeat daily until hair is cleared and lice and eggs are gone.
- Seek homeopathic advice if the scalp has been badly affected. Useful remedies are Oleander, Vinca Minor, Viola Tric, and Pediculosis Capitis.

Hyperactivity

A condition where the child is unable to relax, rest, sleep, or concentrate to the same extent as others of a similar age. There are simple cases of hyperactivity and these are nearly always the manifestation of an allergy. The most common allergens are sugar, wheat products, dairy products, corn, eggs, and nuts. A child can have a mild or severe allergy to one or several foods at the same time. For what to do, see Allergy, page 32.

Hyperventilation

Abnormally rapid breathing that has the effect of reducing the carbon dioxide content of the blood, causing the brain cells to receive less oxygen. This leads to dizziness and even unconsciousness and a lowering of the blood pressure. Hyperventilation may occur in altitude adjustment, some respiratory diseases such as bronchial asthma, anxiety, or for no obvious reason.

WHAT TO DO

The immediate action is to have child breathe with head in a paper bag for 10–20 breaths. This helps to increase the carbon dioxide levels and so restore the oxygen levels to normal. Also attend to the cause.

Penile Infection

Signs of this are swelling, inflammation, pain, and redness, which is worse from urinating. It can be caused by foreign matter collecting under the foreskin and is usually more common where the foreskin is overtight; it can also be caused by a urinary tract infection.

WHAT TO DO—INTERNAL APPLICATION

Golden Seal herb can be taken internally 4–5 times daily for a few days until inflammation subsides.

HOMEOPATHIC

Aconite 30c: Give at first sign for crawling, stinging pain, which comes on suddenly. Urine is red, hot, and painful or difficult to pass.

Cantharis 30c: Raw, burning pain with intolerable urging to urinate. Urine is scalding.

Merc Corr 30c: Penis and testicles are enormously swollen, red, sore, and hot with intense burning on urinating.

WHAT TO DO—EXTERNAL APPLICATIONS

For local redness, use Hypercal lotion to cleanse and disinfect.
SEEK MEDICAL ADVICE if no improvement within twelve hours.

Smelly Feet

Most common causes of smelly feet are undesirable bacteria or fungi, or emotional problems (worry, fear, or anxiety can cause profuse sweating of the feet).

WHAT TO DO

- *Bathe feet:* To water, add a few drops of Pine oil or Witch Hazel tincture to bathe the feet.
- *If emotional,* there are books on Bach Flowers available in most health shops; or seek advice from a natural health practitioner skilled in emotional work or a One Brain or Touch for Health instructor.

Swollen Testicle (Hydrocele)

This is an accumulation of clear, watery, light yellow-colored fluid in the sac around the testicle. It may develop at any age. It is caused by some mild irritation in the lining of the sac. It may occur on both sides but more often only on one. The tendency is for a gradual size increase. There is little or no pain, and it does not seem to affect the general health or be annoying, unless the sac grows to a considerable size.

WHAT TO DO

- The condition may be helped by daily drinks of Golden Seal and Parsley.
- Common homeopathic remedies useful for this condition are Apis, Conium, Graphites, Iodum, Fluoric Acid, or Pulsatilla. The choice will be dependent upon the total symptom picture. See Remedy Pictures, or seek advice from a homeopath.
- Cell salts required for this condition are Calc Fluor and Kali Mur, which can be alternated daily.

Note: Swelling of testicle may also be due to mumps or inguinal hernia. See under these headings.

Undescended Testicles

About two months before birth, the testes descend into the scrotum (the skin-covered bag suspended from the groin). Occasionally, one or both testicles fail to descend. If both, this may lead to sterility in the adult. A good place to check is when the boy is in a warm bath, as the scrotum is relaxed. In cold weather, the testes rise to the top of the scrotum.

WHAT TO DO

- Medically, this condition is corrected by hormone therapy or surgery.
- Homeopathically, Thyroidinum 30c can be effective, especially if the child's development in learning, speech, or physical growth is slow.
- The condition can also be approached from an emotional perspective, especially with the use of Bach Flower essences. The essences and books about them are available in most health shops. Seek advice from a natural health practitioner skilled in emotional work.

Remedy Pictures— Homeopathic

ACONITE

General Characteristics: Mental and physical tension; healthy, strong types who suddenly come down with illness, hemorrhage, visual disturbances, fevers, restlessness, dry hot skin, great thirst, and intolerance of warmth.

Sensations: Tearing, stabbing, cutting pains; numbness and tingling.

Modalities: Worse from exposure to cold, dry winds, drafts, frights, injuries, shocks, operations, evening, night. Better from fresh air.

ANTIMONIUM CRUDUM

General Characteristics: Great sadness, sulky, fretful, cannot bear to be touched or looked at. Gastric disorders worse from overeating. Thick milky white coating on tongue.

Sensations: Loathing of food; very tender feet when walking.

Modalities: Worse from extremes of heat and cold, cold bathing, heat of sun yet can also be better from heat.

ANTIMONIUM TARTUM

General Characteristics: Bad-tempered and complaining worse from consolation and least touch; great drowsiness, cold sweats; great accumulation of mucous, which is difficult to raise; pale, short of breath; heavily coated white tongue; desires, but is worse from apples.

Sensations: Can't raise mucous, can't stand touch, shivering with cold then feverish heat.

Modalities: Worse from heat, cold, damp weather, evening and early night, anger or vexation.

APIS

General Characteristics: Anxiety with restlessness, great drowsiness; edematous swellings; sleep disturbed by pain; anxious dreams with piercing screams during sleep; thirstlessness; complaints right-sided, or right to left.

Sensation: Burning, darting, stinging pains better from cold; sore sensitive skin worse from touch or pressure.

Modalities: Worse from all forms of heat; 4–6 P.M.; sleep.

Do not use before or after Rhus Tox.

ARNICA

General Characteristics: Great fear of being touched; oversensitive to pain; injuries to soft parts; bruises, concussion; offensive discharges with odor of rotten eggs; helps prevent the formation of pus and blood poisoning.

Sensations: Bruised, sore feeling all over; bed feels too hard; head hot, body cold.

Modalities: Worse from rest and lying down. Better from motion.

ARSENICUM ALBUM

General Characteristics: Fastidious, sad, and irritable; fear of death and darkness; great exhaustion yet restless, anxious, and frightened especially during fever. Very chilly. Great thirst for small quantities at frequent intervals. Symptoms recur at regular time intervals.

Sensations: Burning pains better from heat; burning, scant discharges.

Modalities: Worse from cold, damp, midnight to 3 A.M., rest, lying with head low. Better from heat (except the head).

BELLADONNA

General Characteristics: Happy when well, violent symptoms, brain symptoms during illness can become wild delirium, illusions, moaning, jumping out of bed. Sudden local inflammations; fevers with flushed face, throbbing carotids; dry mucous membranes, sparkling eyes.

Sensations: Intolerable sensations, severe throbbing, pain worse lying down, worse from heat. Chilly.

Modalities: Worse from cold, heat of sun, night, least jar, 3 P.M. to 3 A.M., right side. Better from warmth, resting, sitting up, lying on unaffected side.

BRYONIA

General Characteristics: Condition comes on gradually. Irritable. Useful for complaints coming on after suppressed discharges. Excessive dryness of all mucous membranes. Great thirst for large amounts. Constipation, gastric disorders with yellow-coated tongue; right-sided complaints. Lies very still, worse from least movement; worried and maybe delirious; wants to go home.

Sensation: Sharp, stitching pains, worse from motion, better from rest.

Modalities: Worse from slightest motion, at night about 9 P.M. or early A.M., heat of sun. Better from complete mental and physical rest, cool air and applications, lying on painful side.

Do not use before or after Calcarea Carbonica.

CALCAREA CARBONICA

General Characteristics: Slow mental and physical development; anxious, apprehensive; night terrors; slow to learn but tries very hard; difficult teething; easy sweat of head when sleeping; very chilly; sour smelling; enlarged glands.

Sensations: Craves indigestibles, e.g., chalk, dirt, sand; has clammy legs, feet, and hands.

Modalities: Worse from cold and damp, working in water, 2–3 A.M. Better from warmth but not overheating; lying on painful side.

Do not use before or after Bryonia.

CARBO VEGETABILIS

General Characteristics: Lack of reaction to other remedies; extreme weakness after disease, especially due to loss of blood or other body fluids, hemorrhage; injuries; blueness with cold feet and legs, cold sweat, cold breath; very chilly with a hunger for air; excessive accumulation of gas worse upper abdomen, better from passing wind. All food disagrees; very offensive discharges.

Sensations: Burning or painful. Hoarseness and loss of voice worse in damp air and evenings.

Modalities: Worse from overheating. Better from being fanned.

CHAMOMILLA

General Characteristics: Teething problems. Nervous, excitable types who are intolerant and oversensitive to the least pain. Spiteful, irritable, quiet only when carried, impossible to please. One cheek flushed and hot, the other pale and cold. Diarrhea smelling of rotten eggs, worse during teething.

Sensations: Local heat of hands and feet and one cheek; hot discharges, e.g., stools and sweat.

Modalities: Worse from heat, evening, night, teething, sensitive to damp, cold, and wind on ears.

Do not use before or after Nux Vomica.

CHINA

General Characteristics: Very regular recurrence of symptoms, e.g., every second day. Great debility from discharges. Hypersensitive to criticism or touch. Anemic. Excessive flatulence not relieved by belching. Very disturbed digestion.

Sensations: Tearing, drawing pains, bodily soreness worse from rest, better from mild movement. Painlessness of discharges; singing in ears; throbbing, bursting headaches.

Modalities: Worse from cold, damp, autumn, least touch, least draft of air, any mental or physical exertion. Better from warmth and hard pressure.

CINA

Pale-faced children who pick their nose, grind their teeth at night; white discoloration around mouth. Ravenous appetite, bad-tempered, dislikes cuddles. Worm infestations.

COCCULUS

General Characteristics: Cannot bear the least contradiction. Travel sickness with dizziness. Nervous temperaments. Colic not relieved by passing wind.

Sensations: Numbness, parts go to sleep, emptiness in organs, trembling and weakness, feeling of sharp stones in abdomen.

Modalities: Worse from traveling, loss of sleep, fresh air, mental and physical exertion.

DROSERA

Violent spasms, paroxysms of respiratory tract especially during acute illness like measles, whooping cough, etc. Can't get breath from coughing so much. Cough ends in choking, gagging, vomiting, and cold sweat. Constant cough as soon as head touches the pillow. Coughs worse from lying down and after midnight; worse from warmth, drinking, or using the voice.

EUPHRASIA

Profuse, bland discharges from nose with burning discharges from eye. Ailments from injuries especially to eye.
Modalities: Worse in evening or on rising in the morning, indoors, warmth, south wind. Better outdoors.

FERRUM PHOS

First stage of inflammatory processes, e.g., fevers, hemorrhages, etc. Worse 4–6 A.M. and P.M.

GELSEMIUM

General Characteristics: Lethargic, drowsy, dizzy, nervous, and hysterical. Physical complaints arising from nervousness, e.g., diarrhea before exams or new school. Dull headache with blurred vision and dizziness; first stage of fevers with aching back and limbs; chills and absence of thirst; watery discharges; influenza; loss of muscular coordination.
Modalities: Worse when left alone, warm moist weather, emotions, nerves, heat of sun and summer.

HEPAR SULPH

General Characteristics: When conditions show no sign of clearing up. Very chilly. Hypersensitive mentally and physically. Intolerant of pain, touch or draft of air. Sour-smelling excretions; profuse sweats. Use when pus has formed or is about to form; unhealthy skin, staphylococcal infections; injuries often become infected and are very sensitive to drafts or slightest touch. Croup worse from uncovering body parts.

Sensations: Sticking, throbbing pain. Sensation of splinter in throat. Very chilly.

Modalities: Worse from slightest drafts, night. Better from mild, wet weather.

HYPERICUM

General Characteristics: Bad effects of head or spinal injury; pain after injuries or surgery; animal bites or scratches; helps prevent tetanus in puncture wounds.

Sensations: Excessively painful injuries to nerves especially fingers and toes; screaming from slightest motion of neck or arm; pains travel upward; during headache sensation of being lifted up high into the air.

Modalities: Worse from slightest motion of neck or arm; change of weather.

LEDUM

General Characteristics: Always cold, discontented, and peevish. Alternating complaints or symptoms appear diagonally opposite on the body. Helps prevent tetanus; puncture wounds, insect bites, rheumatic, or arthritic complaints.

Sensations: Sticking, tearing, throbbing pain with no heat or swelling rapidly changing locality.

Modalities: Cold, yet worse from warmth of bed. Better from cool applications despite coldness.

LYCOPODIUM

General Characteristics: Intellectually keen types but physically weak, emaciated in upper part of body. Fatigued, forgetful, lacks self-confidence, dislikes company but dreads solitude. Excessive flatulence, craves sweets; constipation predominates; urinary problems; dry skin, especially of palms; dryness of mucous membranes; nose full of crusts or plugs; twitching motion of nostrils.

Sensations: One foot hot the other cold. Right-sided complaints or right to left.

Modalities: Worse from both extremes of temperature but especially heat (except abdomen, which is better from heat); exertion; 4–8 P.M.; sleep. Better from open air, uncovering, gentle motion.

MERCURIUS CORROSIVUS

Acute, violent inflammations, e.g., of eyes, eyelids, kidneys, bowels. Dysentery, appendicitis, peritonitis.

MERCURIUS SOLUBILIS

General Characteristics: Changeable mental states—either slow to answer and despondent, or hurried, anxious, and talkative. Dirty, yellow, rough complexion; violent toothache; weakness and trembling of all limbs; skin eruptions, ulcers, or swollen glands, thin, burning, easy-bleeding discharges that can change to thick yellow/green, bland discharges. Profuse sweat.

Sensations: Intense thirst despite moist tongue. Boring bone pains at night. Bad breath and bad taste in mouth.

Modalities: Worse from heat and cold, at every change especially to damp weather, all night; warmth of bed; lying on right side. Better from resting, high altitudes.

Do not use before or after Silica.

NATRUM MURIATICUM

General characteristics: Anemic, pale, greasy-looking complexions; emaciated about neck, old-looking children;

depressed, emotionally sensitive to music; irritable at small noises; dry skin and mucous membranes or free watery discharges. Mapped tongue with dryness and thirst. Craves salt. Cannot urinate in the presence of others.

Sensations: Must have air but can get chilly.

Modalities: Worse from salt, seaside, company, consolation, heat, especially close rooms, 9–11 A.M. Better from missing meals, being alone, loose clothing.

NATRUM SULPHURICUS

General Characteristics: Depressed, irritable when spoken to. Delirium. Mental as well as physical effects from blow to head. Saddened by music. Greenish-yellow catarrhs, diarrhea on rising and moving about. Loose coughs better by sitting up and holding chest. Asthma.

Sensations: Can have violent, crushing, gnawing pain at base of brain.

Modalities: Worse from all forms of damp; sea air; daytime; lying on left side. Better in the open air.

NUX VOMICA

General characteristics: Irritable, tense, impatient, spiteful, thinks everyone is against them; complaints from too much hard mental work, physically and mentally hypersensitive to pain, criticism, slight ailments. Stomach complaints from too much food causing retching and desire but inability to vomit. Drowsy in evening then wakeful 3–4 A.M. Reawakens at normal time feeling tired and worn out. Must be covered during fevers.

Sensations: Very chilly; great urging but difficult to vomit or pass stool.

Modalities: Worse from drafts, winter, open air, also dry weather. Better from warmth, rest, mild damp weather.

Do not use before or after Chamomilla or Zinc.

PHOSPHORUS

General Characteristics: Quick, lively, sensitive temperaments; rapidly growing, narrow-chested, stoop shouldered, indifferent, disinclined to mental and physical exertion. Slow, depressed yet can be excitable and enthusiastic in fits. Full of fears. Desires sympathy. Fidgety and restless.

Sensations: Burning in spots; intense heat running up back; emptiness. Fear strikes person in stomach. Hunger—must eat often. Craves salt and cold things. Great thirst but can vomit after drinking. Oppressed chest worse using voice, eating, and drinking.

Modalities: Worse from cold (except stomach and head), thunder, weather changes, twilight to midnight, lying left side. Better from lying down and sleeping.

Do not use before or after Causticum.

PULSATILLA

General Characteristics: Gentle, yielding, unstable emotional temperament. Anemic, pale-faced. Great changeableness of symptoms, shifting locality and sensation. Tearful, self-pity. Loves consolation. Can be submissive or obstinate, easily upset. Changeable stools. Digestive complaints from overloading with rich, fatty foods. White-coated tongue. Sleepless early evening but sleeps late into morning. Copious greenish-yellow thick, bland discharges.

Sensations: Thirstlessness despite dry mouth. Chilliness despite being better in cool air.

Modalities: Worse from warm rooms, twilight to midnight, lying on left or painless side. Better from gentle motion in cool, open air despite feeling chilly.

PYROGENIUM

Septic blood conditions when other remedies fail to permanently improve. Horribly offensive excretions; tongue fiery red, clean, and smooth. Very rapid pulse. Very restless and sore in bed. Complete inertia of bowel.

Sensations: Complains of bed being too hard; sweet but very foul taste in mouth.

RHUS TOXICENDRON

General Characteristics: Pains worse during rest and on beginning to move, yet better from continued motion; very restless during fevers with red, dry, cracked tongue and triangular red tip. Sad, apprehensive, tearful worse at night. Acrid, foul secretions and excretions. Usually worse right side. Sprains and strains. Acute skin diseases. Conditions brought on by overexertion.

Modalities: Worse from cold, wet weather, cold winds, getting wet especially after overheating; before storms, during and after rest. Better from warm applications; during warm weather.

Do not use before or after Apis.

RUTA GRAVEOLENS

General Characteristics: Mechanical injuries of bones; sprains, flat feet, overstrained eyes.

Sensations: Bruised pain, lameness; burning, aching, strained eyes.

Modalities: Worse from cold, wet weather, lying on painful part, outdoors, reading, or straining eyes. Better from warmth and moving about indoors.

SEPIA

General Characteristics: Indifferent even to family. Melancholy worse from consolation and company. Tearful, disinclined to mental and physical labor. Hypersensitive to and irritated by noise and music. Constipation. Bed wetting. Easy sweating between folds of skin. Hair falls out.

Sensations: Chilly. Sinking feeling at 11 A.M. not better by eating. Nausea at smell of food. Hates fats. Itching not better by scratching.

Modalities: Worse from stuffy rooms, before thunder, moist hot weather, excitement, milk. Better from violent exertion.

Do not use before or after Lachesis.

SILICA

General Characteristics: Lack of vital heat, icy coldness, light, fine types with dry skin, pale face, large sweaty heads. Nervous, anxious, timid but irritable if aroused. Melancholy, desires consolation. Lacks self-confidence yet gets through by sheer effort of will. Obstinate, headstrong, but cries with gentle treatment. Hypersensitive to noise. Slow learning to walk; weak ankles; sleep walkers. Long-lasting suppurations, streptococcal infections; bad effects of vaccination; ingrowing toenails; unhealthy, easily infected skin.

Sensations: Coldness from neck up over head to one eye, worse from draft and uncovering, better from wrapping up warmly. Stitching, stabbing, sticking pains worse from motion. Offensive foot sweat. Clammy hands and feet.

Modalities: Worse from cold, approach of winter, new and waxing moon. Better from warmth, wrapping head up warmly, summer, humid weather.

Do not use before or after Mercurius.

SULPHUR

General Characteristics: Untidy, sedentary types, intolerant of bathing and covering, grumblers; variable hunger and thirst; can eat a lot and stay thin; likes sweets. Internal problems caused by suppressed skin eruptions. Relapsing conditions; lack of reaction to remedies in acute diseases.

Skin eruptions worse from warmth and washing. Smelly eruptions and discharges.

Sensations: Scratching causes burning. Hands and feet burning hot in bed.

Modalities: Worse from heat, warmth of bed, standing still, bathing. Better from cold air.

THUJA

General Characteristics: Ailments from vaccination, especially diarrhea. Depressed, dislikes company, quarrelsome, loss of memory, always hurried. Decayed roots of teeth. Greasy complexion, especially forehead. Unhealthy skin. Green, offensive, catarrhal discharges. Constipation or sudden, gurgling diarrhea. Overgrowths of tissues, e.g., warts, moles, sties. Sweats only on uncovered parts or all over except head especially while sleeping. Deformed, brittle nails.

Sensations: Strange, fixed ideas (of something alive in abdomen; of soul and body being separated; of limbs being made of glass; of domination by a superior being).

Modalities: Worse from damp, cold air, bathing, heat of bed, A.M. and throughout day or after 3 A.M. and 3 P.M. Better from scratching, stretching, after sweating.

Remedy Pictures—Cell Salts

CALC FLUOR

Found in surface of bones, tooth enamel, and in elastic fibers of skin, muscular tissue, and blood vessels. Deficiency causes relaxed tissues and elastic fibers, e.g. unnaturally loose teeth, varicose veins, or hemorrhoids.

Modalities: Worse from damp. Better from rubbing and applications to affected parts.

CALC PHOS

Found in bones, teeth, connective tissue, blood, and gastric juice. Deficiency causes slow teething, anemia, bone diseases, poor digestion.

Modalities: Worse from cold, motion, getting wet, change of weather. Better from rest, warmth, lying down.

CALC SULPH

Found in skin, cells, and blood. Deficiency causes slow healing of wounds, excessive formation of pus—catarrh, boils, ulcers, abscesses, pimples. Pus is thick, yellow, and sometimes blood-streaked.

Modalities: Worse from getting wet, washing, or working in water.

FERR PHOS

Found in blood. Deficiency causes fever, inflammation, poor appetite, weight loss. Tongue clean, red, inflamed, or swollen.

Modalities: Worse from motion. Better from cold.

KALI MUR

Found in blood, nerve cells, and muscles. Deficiency causes glandular swellings, liver troubles. Thick, white, sticky discharge. Tongue has white-gray coating. Ulcers, blisters on tongue.

Modalities: Worse motion; rich, fatty foods.

KALI PHOS

Found especially in brain and nerves; also in muscle and blood. Deficiency causes irritability, fearfulness, exhaustion. Tongue brown or mustard-colored, dry or inflamed; breath is offensive.

Modalities: Worse from noise, physical, or mental exertion, cold air, beginning movement after rest. Better from gentle motion, eating, rest, excitement.

KALI SULPH

Carries oxygen to cells of skin and mucous membranes. Deficiency causes lack of oxygen in skin with resultant chilliness and desire for fresh air. Especially useful in later stages of inflammation where discharges are yellow, slimy, sticky, or greenish. Tongue is yellow and slimy. Loss of taste.

Modalities: Worse from warm room; toward evening. Better from cool, fresh air.

MAG PHOS

Found in nerves and muscles. Deficiency causes cramps, spasms, convulsions, toothache, sharp shooting pains. Especially indicated in lean, thin people with highly nervous temperaments.

Modalities: Worse from touch, cold wind, washing. Better from application of heat, firm pressure, friction, and bending double.

NAT MUR

Found in every liquid and solid part of the body. Acts upon the lymphatic system, blood, liver, spleen, mucous lining of alimentary canal. Deficiency causes fluid imbalance, e.g., bloated skin or excessively dry skin. Loss of taste or salty taste. Frothy saliva. Failure to respond to other cell salts.

Modalities: Worse from seaside, cold weather, morning.

NAT PHOS

Found in blood, muscles, nerve cells, brain cells, and intercellular fluids. Deficiency causes excess acidity in system, worms, gastric disturbances from overfeeding on milk and sugar. Coppery or acidic taste in mouth. Sour-smelling discharge. Tongue thick, yellow moist coating.

Modalities: Worse afternoon or evening.

NAT SULPH

Found in intercellular fluid. Regulates quantity of water in body and eliminates excessive fluids. Deficiency causes swollen skin, liver diseases, bilious conditions. Tongue dirty greenish-yellow coating. Bitter taste in mouth.

Modalities: Worse from using water, living in low damp places, wet weather, eating watery plants, fish. Better from dry warm atmosphere.

SILICA

Found in blood, bile, skin, hair, nails, bones, nerves, and glands. Deficiency causes slow formation of pus. Chilly sensitive people. Festering sores. Ulcers on tongue. Offensive thick yellow discharges.

Modalities: Worse from cold. Better warm rooms, warm applications.

Bibliography

Airola, Paavo. *How to Get Well.* Phoenix, AZ: Health Plus Publications, 1974.

Blackmore, M. C. H. *Mineral Deficiencies in Human Cells.* Sydney, Australia. Blackmore's Communications Service, 1983.

Boericke, Dr. William. *Materia Medica and Repertory.* New Delhi, India: Jain Publications, 1982.

Borland, Douglas M. *Homoeopathy for Mother and Infant.* London: British Homeopathic Association,

Chapman, J. B. *Dr. Schuessler's Biochemistry.* Northhamptonshire, England: Thorsons Publishers, Ltd., 1973.

Fishbein, M.D., Morris. *The Handy Home Medical Adviser.* New York: Doubleday, 1952.

Gibson, Dr. D. M. *Homoeopathy: First Aid in Accidents and Ailments.* London: British Homoeopathy Association, 1977.

Green, Dr. Christopher. *Toddler Taming.* New York: Fawcett Columbine, 1985.

Kent, J. T. *Repertory of the Homeopathic Materia Medica.* New Delhi, India: Jain Publications, 1985.

Kichlu and Bose. *Descriptive Medicine.* Reprint, New Delhi, India: Jain Publications, 1984.

Lautie, Raymond, D.Sc., and Passeberg, Andres M.D. *Aromatherapy.* Northhamptonshire, England: Thorsons Publishers, Ltd., 1979.

Leavitt, Sheldon, M.D. *Homeopathic Therapeutics as Applied to Obstetrics.* Calcutta, India: A. P. Homeopathic Library, 1962.

Lust, John. *The Herb Book.* New York: Bantam Books, 1974.

New Zealand Health Department. *Health & Development Record.*

Pàlos, Stephan. *The Chinese Art of Healing.* Toronto, Canada: Bantam, 1972.

Parker, Merren. *For Goodness Sake.* Auckland, New Zealand: Collins, 1978.

Schuessler, Dr. W. H. *Biochemic Pocket Guide.* New Delhi, India: Pratap Medical Publishers.

Shepherd, Dr. Dorothy. *Homoeopathy in Epidemic Diseases.* Reprint, New Delhi, India: Jain Publications, 1967, 1983.

Speight, Leslie. *Homoeopathy and Immunisation.* Essex, England: Health Science Press, 1983.

Speight, Phyllis. *Homeopathic Remedies for Children.* Essex, England: Health Science Press, 1983.

St. Johns Ambulance First Aid Association & Brigade. *First Aid Manual.* Reed Methuen, 1972.

Woods, Dr. H. Fergie. *Homeopathic Treatment in the Nursery.* London: British Homoeopathy Association.

Suppliers of Natural Remedies

Natural remedies are easily obtained from health shops and some pharmacists. Their suppliers have mailing systems, so that you can order directly if you have difficulty obtaining remedies locally.

United States Homeopathic Suppliers
Arrowroot Standard Direct, Ltd.
83 East Lancaster Ave.
Paoli, PA 19301
Tel: (800) 234-8879
customerservice@arrowroot.com

Heel, Inc.
11600 Cochiti S.E.
Albuquerque, NM 87123
Tel: (800) 621-7644
Fax: (505) 275-1672

HealthCo Northwest
170 West Ellendale
Dallas, OR 97338
Tel: (503) 831-0871

Toll free: (888) 715-6398
Fax: (503) 831-0873
dockperson@aol.com

The Hickory Chemist
888 2nd Ave.
New York, NY 10017
Tel: (212) 223-6333

Homeopathy Works
124 Fairfax Street
Berkeley Springs, WV 25411
Tel: (304) 258-2541

Longevity Pure Medicines
9595 Wilshire Blvd. #706
Beverly Hills, CA 90212
Tel: (800) 327-5519
Fax: (508) 892-1896

Mediral International, Inc.
5260 East 39th Ave.
Denver, CO 80207
Toll free: (877) 633-4725
Tel: (303) 331-6161
Fax: (303) 355-4155
info@mediral.com

Newton Homeopathic
Laboratories, Inc.
2360 Rockaway Industrial Blvd.
Conyers, GA 30207
Toll free: (800) 448-7256
Tel: (770) 922-2644
info line: (800) NOSODE 3
toll free fax: (800)760-5550
mailinfo@newtonlabs.net

Santa Monica Homeopathic
Pharmacy
629 Broadway (at 7th St.)
Santa Monica, CA 90401
Tel: (310) 395-1131
Fax: (310) 395-7861
smhomeopahic@hotmail.com

UTC/Bengal Allen
512 1st Ave.
East Bradenton, FL 34208
Tel: (941) 748-5114

Washington Homeopathic
Products, Inc.
4915 Del Ray Ave.
Bethesda, MD 20814
Toll free: (800) 336-1695
Tel: (301) 656-1695
Fax: (310) 656-1847

United States Herbal Suppliers
Horizon Herbs, LLC
PO Box 69
Williams, OR 97544
Tel: (541) 846-6704
Fax: (541) 846-6233

The Wellness Store
13300 Bothell Highway, #6129
Mill Creek, WA 98012
Tel: (425) 750-5490
Fax: (425) 750-5490
leaflady@leaflady.org

Australasian College of Herbal
Studies Apothecary Shoppe
530 First Ave.
PO Box 57
Lake Oswego, OR 97034
Toll free: (800) 635-6652
Tel: (503) 487-8839

Planet Herb
PO Box 130
Rt. 219 North
Renick, WV 24966
Toll free: (888) 480-4372
www.planetherb.com

Monterey Spice Company
719 Swift St.
Suite 106
Santa Cruz, CA 95060
Toll free: (800) 500-6148
Fax: (831) 426-2792

Samara Botane
1811 Queen Anne Ave. North, #103
Seattle, WA 898109
Tel: (206) 283-7191
www.wingseed.com

Frontier Herbs
Friends from the Earth
667 CR 500 East
Chandlerville, IL 62627
nvenzon@casscomm.com
www.friendsfromtheearth.com

Viable Herbal Solutions
PO Box 969
Morrisville, PA 19067
Toll free: (800) 505-9475
Tel: (215) 337-8182
Toll free fax: (800) 505-9476
Fax: (215) 505-8186
viable@voicenet.com

Glenbrook Farm Herbs and Such
15922 76th St.
Live Oak, FL 32060
Tel: (808) 716-7627
Fax: (904) 362-5321

Maggie's Herb Basket
141 Main St.
Landisville, PA 17538
Tel: (717) 898-6334
Fax: (717) 898-6117

Index

A

abdomen, 3, 36, 51, 94, 112, 130, 161, 187, 191, 203, 228
abrasions, 30, 228–29
abscess, 27–28, 52–53, 174, 209, 257
accidents, car, 109, 113
aches, 32, 81, 124, 149, 174, 182, 198, 253
adenoids, 130, 131, 216
AIDS (Acquired Immune Deficiency Syndrome), 29–32
airways, 44, 61, 72–73, 109, 115, 128, 172
allergy, 32–34, 35, 47, 91, 94, 95, 106, 132, 143–44, 169, 171, 195, 202, 214, 239
anemia, 35–38, 164, 172, 247, 250, 252, 256
antibiotics, x, 34, 81, 91, 143, 175, 214, 221
anus, 51, 79, 80, 107, 129, 142, 154, 155, 227, 228
anxiety, 3, 10, 29, 36, 38–42, 50, 63, 85, 88, 91, 95, 106, 108, 115, 123, 153, 154, 164, 165, 171, 173, 175, 180, 195, 196, 199, 201, 239, 240, 244, 246, 250, 254. *See also* stress
appendicitis, 42–44, 250
artificial respiration, 31, 61, 109–10, 177
asphyxia, 61, 115
asthma, 2, 32, 44–48, 61, 82, 239, 251

B

babies, 49–52, 79, 89, 91–92, 135, 145, 152–56, 165, 202, 203, 207–8, 213–15

back, backache, 3, 37, 138, 148, 164, 187, 203, 204, 210, 220, 221, 248
bacteria, 34, 35, 91, 92, 93, 94, 105, 160, 193, 240
bad breath, 56, 97, 99, 101, 103, 130, 134, 140, 149, 155, 165, 167, 208, 209, 236, 250, 257
bed-wetting, 32, 40, 87, 89, 253
bee sting, 54, 57, 143
behavioral disorders, 32, 38–42, 244, 247
belching, 36, 46, 88, 96, 97, 142, 154, 155, 180, 247
belly button, 42, 51, 141
birth, birthmarks, 30, 41, 50, 51
bites, 8, 30, 32, 53–57, 202, 210, 249
bleeding, 51, 79, 111–12, 127, 146, 165, 183, 195, 203, 204, 207, 208, 209, 214, 223, 228, 229–30, 232, 236. *See also* menstruation
blisters, 32, 58, 66, 68, 70, 75–76, 116, 145, 166, 170, 179, 180, 202, 203, 236, 257
blood poisoning, 145
blows, 117–18, 134–35, 251
boils, 58–60, 103, 174, 257
bowels, 43, 107, 123, 137, 142, 153, 155, 158, 165, 167, 175, 220, 250, 251, 253. *See also* constipation; diarrhea
brain, 116, 124, 134–35, 199, 245, 251
breasts, breast feeding, 51, 52–53, 129, 130, 164, 168, 215

breathing difficulties, 3, 35, 37, 44, 45, 50, 54, 60–62, 63, 72–73, 75, 80, 82, 83, 84, 85, 86, 97, 98, 99, 109–11, 115, 125, 128, 130, 136, 142, 160, 172, 174, 175, 176, 177, 180, 181, 195, 211, 224, 226, 233, 239, 244, 248. *See also* obstruction

bronchitis, 32, 61, 62–65, 71, 82, 102, 151, 185

bruises, 7, 8, 14, 50, 51, 52, 65, 205, 229, 232, 244, 253

burns, 7, 66–69, 195, 210

C

Candida Albicans, 34, 107, 213–15. *See also* thrush

car sickness. *See* travel sickness

casualty care, 109–13

catarrh, 36, 101, 104, 155, 156, 166, 196, 197, 198, 236, 251, 255, 257

cell salts, 3, 15–16, 17, 18, 23, 39

chemicals, 19, 20, 32, 129, 152, 160, 177, 179

chest, 4, 8, 62, 63, 73, 83, 84, 111–12, 149, 159, 174, 175, 176, 186, 187, 203, 204, 213

chicken pox, 22, 23, 70–72, 202

choking, 72–73, 85, 248

chorea, 185

circulation, 21, 66, 83–84, 110, 113, 135, 186, 210, 218

colds, 4, 6–7, 22, 47, 62, 64, 74–75, 81, 82, 85, 101, 102, 118, 122, 129, 133, 145, 148, 169, 174, 196, 212

cold sores, 75–76, 166

colic, 49, 50, 93, 94, 95, 96, 142, 164, 173, 174, 211

collapse, 115, 178, 180

coma, 3, 87, 89, 113. *See also* unconsciousness

compress, 7, 43, 52, 57, 91, 94, 117, 216, 230

concussion, 134, 135, 244

congestion, 44, 46, 47, 74, 102, 103, 129, 149, 164, 169–71, 180, 187, 198, 212

conjunctiva, conjunctivitis, 77–78, 152–56

constipation, 35, 37, 42, 43, 47, 51, 78–80, 88, 89, 90, 94, 123, 133, 134, 140, 153, 154, 163, 164, 165, 245, 250, 253, 255

convulsions, 3, 113, 122, 124–26, 137, 160, 161, 162, 177, 180, 181, 207, 210, 225, 226, 258

cough, 3, 37, 42, 43, 45, 46, 61, 62, 63, 64, 74, 75, 80–82, 84, 85, 97, 141, 148, 149, 157, 158, 159, 166, 175, 176, 182, 194, 224–26, 248, 251

CPR (Cardio-Pulmonary Resuscitation), 110–11, 115

cradle cap, 49

cramps, 61, 83–84, 93, 95, 97, 136, 137, 142, 163, 164, 165, 178, 210, 221, 258

croup, 62, 82, 84–86, 249

cuts, 30, 121, 174, 210, 228–29, 232, 236

cystitis, 32, 220–22

D

debility, 187, 226, 247. *See also* weakness

dehydration, 3, 62, 91, 93, 132, 225

delirium, 136, 137, 159, 160, 161, 178, 194, 245, 251

depression, 18, 32, 37, 40, 41, 53, 89, 137, 138, 140, 148, 149, 150, 155, 164, 165, 181, 194, 243, 244, 251, 252, 255

dermatitis, contact, 202, 236–37

development, slow, 41–42, 246

diabetes, juvenile, 87–89, 113

diaper rash, 51, 89–90, 202

diarrhea, 32, 35, 36, 38, 43, 51, 80, 90–94, 97, 136, 138, 139, 143, 153, 155, 159, 164, 179, 181, 195, 196, 207, 215, 246, 248, 251, 255

diet, 15, 19–20, 34, 35–36, 43, 62, 78–79, 87–88, 92, 94–95, 149, 154, 183, 185–86, 193–94, 216

digestive problems, 20, 21, 34, 35, 36, 94–97, 132, 138, 149, 152, 173, 174, 199, 218, 236, 243, 245, 247, 251, 252, 256, 258. *See also* allergy

diphtheria, 22, 23, 62, 97–99, 166

discharge, 28, 47, 60, 77–78, 82, 108, 118, 119, 145, 146, 149, 169–71, 193, 196, 197, 198, 203, 211, 214,

231, 244, 245, 246, 247, 248, 250, 251, 257, 258, 259

dizziness, 36, 37, 56, 62, 83, 124, 133, 135, 139, 162, 180, 232, 239, 247, 248

dog bite, 53–54

drowsiness, 113, 136, 155, 156, 160, 168, 178, 194, 200, 244, 248, 251. *See also* fatigue; tiredness

drugs, xi, xii, 18, 19, 31–32, 137, 143, 152, 177

E

earache, 32, 102, 103, 104, 105, 158, 159, 160, 173, 195, 218, 219

ears, xi, 3, 32, 36, 37, 90, 100, 101–6, 107, 128, 129, 130, 135, 157, 159, 160, 166, 193, 195, 203, 210, 216, 218, 247

eczema, 8, 32, 90, 106–8, 183, 202

electricity, 67, 69, 109

emergency techniques, 54–55, 108–16

emotions, emotional disorders, 38–41, 106, 133, 163, 164, 165, 248, 251, 252

encephalitis, 157

epilepsy, 113, 125

Eustachian tube, blocked, 101, 103

exhaustion, 36, 37, 41, 42, 46, 50, 52, 73, 92, 99, 137, 148, 154, 155, 180, 187, 194, 224, 226, 244, 257

eyes, 3, 10, 32, 37, 51, 65, 74, 75, 87, 116–21, 123, 124, 133, 134, 136, 137, 138, 140, 149, 150, 152, 153, 157, 158, 159, 160, 161, 162, 179, 180, 189, 195, 197, 198, 203, 211, 228, 245, 248, 250, 253

F

fainting, faintness, 36, 73, 96, 115, 136, 164, 172, 195, 219, 232

fatigue, 60, 81, 185, 186, 249. *See also* drowsiness; tiredness

fear, 32, 91, 115, 116, 123, 134, 141, 161, 164, 180, 182, 196, 199, 200, 201, 224, 240, 244, 252, 257

feet, 63, 87, 129, 162, 183, 186, 191, 203, 240, 243, 253, 254, 255

fever, 37, 42, 43, 58, 61, 62, 63, 64, 70, 71, 74, 75, 76, 85, 93, 97, 99, 122–25, 126, 129, 130, 135, 137, 138, 139, 148, 149, 150, 151, 153, 154, 157, 158, 159, 160, 161, 162, 164, 166, 167, 168, 171, 174, 175, 176, 181, 186, 187, 189, 190, 193, 194, 198, 200, 210, 211, 213, 215, 216, 224, 243, 245, 248, 253, 257

first aid, 3. *See also* emergency techniques

fits, 3, 38, 122, 124–26

flatulence, 32, 35, 95, 96, 142, 154, 174, 246, 247, 250

flea bite, 54, 57

flu. *See* influenza

flushing, 164, 204, 245

food poisoning, 179, 180–81

fractures, 3, 111–12, 113, 126–28, 135, 210, 230

fright, 50, 93, 125, 163, 199, 243, 245

frostbite, 115

fungus, 160, 187–88, 213–15, 240

G

gallstones, 152, 155

gangrene, 87

gastroenteritis, 94, 95. *See also* digestive problems

genitals, 164, 191, 214, 215, 220, 227, 239–40

German measles, 22, 23, 129, 189–90, 203

giddiness, 35, 195

glands, 28, 56, 58, 59, 64, 75, 99, 103, 104, 105, 129–31, 148, 152, 159, 160, 166, 168, 173, 189, 190, 194, 203, 213, 215–18, 225, 246, 250, 257. *See also* lymphatic system

glaucoma, 117, 121

groin, 130, 187, 203

growing pains, 237

gums, 165, 208, 209, 214, 215, 236

H

hay fever. *See* allergy

head, 113, 134–35, 146, 174, 182, 187, 196, 197, 198, 203, 208, 237–38, 244, 249, 254

headache, 32, 35, 37, 38, 80, 81, 99, 119, 120, 121, 124, 132–34, 136, 137, 138, 140, 148, 150, 159, 160,

161, 162, 163, 164, 168, 170, 174,
181, 186, 189, 193, 194, 196, 198,
200, 204, 215, 220, 247, 248, 249
health kits, 2, 6, 10, 80
hearing difficulties, 100, 101, 103
heartbeat, 46, 110, 111, 113, 122, 177,
185, 186. *See also* pulse
heartburn, 35, 94, 95, 96, 141, 142
heart disorders, 18, 98, 185, 186, 195, 213
heat exhaustion, heatstroke, 135–37
hemorrhage, 35, 36, 52, 115, 116, 229,
243, 246, 248. *See also* bleeding
hemorrhoids, 79, 80, 256
hepatitis, 9, 22, 23, 94, 137–40, 152
herbs, 4–8, 17, 20, 39, 49, 52, 71, 147
hernia, 140–42, 241
herpes, 70, 75
hiccups, 51, 97
hives, 32, 143–44, 202
HIV (Human Immunodeficiency Virus),
29–32
Hodgkin's disease, 129
homeopathy, 3, 9–14, 17–18, 21–22,
23, 39, 47, 49–51, 52
hormones, 162, 241
hyperactivity, 32, 238–39
hypersensitivity, 33, 40, 106, 162, 165,
244, 246, 247, 248, 251, 253, 254.
See also allergy
hyperventilation, 38, 62, 239

I
immune system, 19–24, 29, 31, 32, 99,
147, 148. *See also* resistance
immunization, 21, 22–24. *See also* vaccination
impetigo, 145–46, 191, 203
influenza, 4, 22, 23, 40, 81, 94, 132,
148–51, 169, 248
insects, 10, 32, 105, 143, 144, 249
insomnia, 38, 63, 89, 102, 154,
198–200, 238–39, 247, 251, 252
irritability, 10, 35, 40, 41, 50, 51, 53, 70,
71, 87, 96, 102, 139, 155, 159, 160,
163, 164, 165, 167, 170, 171, 227,
228, 244, 245, 246, 251, 253, 254,
257
itching, 8, 32, 54, 57, 70, 71, 76, 89, 90,
103, 104, 105, 106, 107, 108, 138,

140, 143, 146, 152, 153, 154, 155,
159, 164, 170, 179, 183, 184, 188,
191–92, 202, 203, 214, 215, 227,
228, 236, 238, 254

J
jaundice, 9, 51, 138, 140, 152–56
jaw spasm, 167, 210–11
jellyfish sting, 54, 55

K
kidney disorders, 3, 21, 35, 78, 87, 160,
173, 213, 216, 220, 250

L
lacerations, 229
lactose intolerance, 9–10, 214. *See also*
milk allergy
laryngitis, 84–86
learning difficulties, 38–42, 246
lethargy, 160, 164, 182, 248
leukemia, 129
lice, head, 146, 237–38
ligaments, 65, 173, 204–6
limbs, 50, 124, 127, 129, 135, 137,
138, 148, 150, 153, 157, 159, 181,
189, 193, 201, 202, 203, 204–6,
211, 248, 250, 255
liver, 9, 21, 78, 133, 137–40, 152, 183,
236, 257, 258, 259
lockjaw, 210–11
lungs, 21, 44, 45, 47, 61, 62, 78, 80, 86,
98, 109–10, 153, 157, 172, 174–77
lymphatic system, 21, 42, 78, 129–31,
167, 197, 203, 213, 258

M
malaria, 135
mastoiditis, 102
measles, 22, 23, 82, 94, 102, 132,
157–60, 169, 176, 189, 190, 203,
225, 248
medications. *See* drugs
meningitis, 22, 23, 41, 102, 125, 158,
160–62
menstruation, 36, 37, 162–65
metabolism, faulty, 32–33, 42, 87–89,
91, 183
miasms, 14, 24

migraine, 132
milk allergy, 19, 29, 50, 51, 52, 53, 63, 95, 97. *See also* lactose intolerance
miscarriage, 210
mites, 191, 192
mosquito bite, 54, 57
mothers, nursing, 52–53, 91–92
mouth, 3, 40, 72, 88, 96, 125, 129, 143, 145, 157, 161, 165–66, 170, 177, 178, 189, 203, 204, 209, 210, 213, 216, 247, 252
mucous, 3, 12, 19, 37, 44, 46, 47, 62, 63, 64, 74, 75, 80, 81, 82, 100, 104, 170, 174, 176, 196, 197, 216, 224, 225, 244
mucous membranes, 35, 36, 169, 198, 213–15, 245, 250, 251
mumps, xii, 22, 23, 104, 129, 166–68, 241
muscles, 33, 65, 83–84, 88, 120, 124, 126, 132, 136, 140–42, 149, 162, 173, 174, 200, 204–6, 210, 211, 229, 236, 248

N

nails, 38, 39, 40, 255
nausea, 42, 46, 88, 94, 95, 96, 97, 99, 132, 133, 136, 137, 138, 139, 142, 155, 159, 162, 164, 174, 178, 179, 181, 218–19, 225, 226, 254
navel, 42, 51, 141
neck, 3, 153, 160, 168, 189, 204, 210, 211, 249. *See also* glands
nephritis, 193, 195
nerves, nervousness, 38, 66, 88, 89, 93, 95, 98, 113, 123, 124–26, 127, 134, 155, 160, 165, 173, 182, 184, 199, 200, 201, 209, 211, 218, 229, 246, 247, 248, 249, 254, 258
nightmares, 37, 40, 200–201, 228, 244, 246
nipples, 52, 53, 107
nose, 18, 19, 51, 62, 74, 75–76, 97–99, 145, 148, 149, 150, 157, 163, 164, 169–72, 180, 189, 190, 197, 198, 203, 216, 224, 225
nosodes, homeopathic, xii, 21–22, 23, 71, 93, 167, 176, 182, 226
numbness, 56, 116, 133, 182, 205, 232, 243, 247

O

obstruction, 42, 61, 62, 72–73, 86, 105, 109, 112, 121, 125, 172, 229–30, 233
oxygen, lack of, 61, 115, 175, 239, 257–58

P

pain, 27, 28, 32, 35, 39, 40, 42, 43, 50, 51, 52, 53, 56, 57, 58, 59, 60, 62, 63, 64, 65, 66, 68, 73, 79, 81, 82, 92, 94, 95, 96, 97, 99, 113, 116, 117, 119, 120, 121, 123, 127–28, 129, 130, 131, 138, 139, 141, 142, 147, 149, 150, 155, 161, 162, 163, 164, 165, 166, 167, 168, 173–74, 176, 178, 179, 180, 181, 185, 186, 187, 189, 195, 196, 197, 198, 204, 205, 207–9, 210, 211, 216, 220, 221, 231–32, 236, 237, 239–40, 243, 245, 246, 247, 248, 249, 250, 251, 253, 254, 258
pallor, 10, 35, 37, 172, 180, 195, 196, 204, 226, 228, 233, 244, 247, 250, 252, 254
palpitations, 35, 37, 38, 41, 73, 149, 175. *See also* pulse
pancreas, 87–89
paralysis, 181–82, 211
parasites, 35, 93, 146, 191, 227–28, 237–38
penis, 191, 239–40
period, menstrual, 162–65
peritonitis, 42–44, 250
phobias, 38, 39–40, 41
pimples, 131, 202, 236, 257
pleurisy, 185
pneumonia, 22, 62, 82, 94, 149, 158, 174–77, 185, 193, 195, 210, 225
poisoning, 54–57, 62, 113, 137, 176, 177–81
poliomyelitis (polio), 22, 24, 181–82
poultice, 7, 27, 52, 59, 65, 141, 205
pregnancy, 34, 83, 87, 152, 163, 190, 210
psoriasis, 90, 183–84, 203
pulse rate, 33, 35, 42, 50, 61, 110, 111, 115, 123, 124, 135, 136, 137, 150, 153, 178, 180, 187, 195, 196, 198, 233, 253

pus, 27, 28, 58, 60, 69, 105, 118, 131, 145, 146, 147, 151, 196, 203, 217, 232, 236, 238, 244, 249, 257, 259

R

rash, 32, 70, 143–44, 157, 158, 159, 179, 189, 193, 194, 201–4, 218
rat bite, rat poison, 57, 177
Recovery Position, 111, 125, 177, 195–96
rectum, 142, 154. *See also* anus
remedies, 2–3, 9–14, 17–18, 183, 218
Remedy Pictures, 3, 10, 12, 13, 23, 243–59
resistance, 19–24, 74, 99, 138, 150. *See also* immune system
respiratory tract, 62, 76, 84–86, 148, 160, 210, 225, 236, 239, 248
resuscitation, 177, 180. *See also* artificial respiration; CPR (Cardio-Pulmonary Resuscitation)
rheumatic fever, 174, 185–87, 193, 195, 213, 216
Rh factor incompatibility, 153
RICE Formula, 204
ringworm, 187–88, 203
Rubella, 189–90, 203. *See also* German measles

S

scabies, 191–92, 203
scalp, 49, 129, 183, 184, 187, 203, 238
scarlet fever, 22, 24, 94, 129, 193–95, 204
schizophrenia, 32
scratches, 249
screaming, 161, 200, 249
seasickness. *See* travel sickness
septicemia, 145
sexually transmitted diseases (STDs), 31
shellfish allergy, 94
shingles, 70
shock, 3, 50, 52, 62, 66, 67, 68, 109, 113, 116, 117, 127, 134, 136, 164, 195–96, 229, 231, 243
sinus, sinusitis, 32, 132, 160, 170, 193, 195, 196–98, 236. *See also* congestion
skin, 3, 8, 32, 35, 37, 45, 50, 51, 53, 56, 61, 73, 78, 86, 88, 89, 111, 115, 123, 125, 126, 136, 137, 138, 140,

152–56, 161, 164, 174, 178, 179, 180, 181, 185, 186, 192, 194, 195, 196, 202, 205, 226, 232, 243, 246, 250, 251, 253, 254, 258, 259. *See also* itching; *specific skin ailments*
sleep, 125, 134, 135, 153, 161, 198–201, 244. *See also* insomnia
sleepwalking, 41, 200, 254
smallpox, 129, 210
snake venom, 35, 54–55
sneezing, 42, 63, 74, 81, 149, 150, 157, 166, 170, 197, 198, 224
sores, xi, 3, 7, 14, 30, 145–46, 191. *See also* ulcers
spasm, 45, 67, 81, 82, 83–84, 97, 121, 142, 161, 162, 164, 165, 179, 210, 211, 220, 221, 224–26, 248, 258
spine, 47, 94, 111, 116, 132, 181–82, 211, 249
spleen, 152, 154
sprains, 7, 174, 204–6, 232, 253
squinting, 120–21, 228
stings, 53–57, 143, 179
stomach, stomachache, 3, 36, 38, 94, 95, 141, 142, 158, 160, 173, 178, 180, 181, 200, 225
strains, 7, 174, 204–6, 253
strep throat, 213
stress, 31, 32, 33, 34, 47, 48, 54, 60, 94, 96, 132, 165, 185, 186, 195, 200, 207–8. *See also* anxiety
stroke, 113, 116
sty, 118–19, 255
sucking difficulties, 12, 13, 16, 50, 53
sugar, in blood, 87, 88, 132, 133
sunburn, sunstroke, 67, 69, 116, 135
surgery, pain after, 249
swallowing difficulties, 56, 95, 99, 130, 162, 167, 210, 211, 215, 217

T

tantrums, 38–39, 40
tears, tear duct, 29, 118, 119
teeth, teething, 84, 93, 96, 109, 146, 161, 173, 196, 207–9, 227, 228, 236, 246, 247, 250, 255, 256, 258
temperature, 69, 74, 115, 135, 136, 147, 148, 199, 203, 220, 250. *See also* fever

tendons, 65, 204–6, 229
testicles, 168, 240, 241–42
tetanus, 22, 24, 210–12, 231, 232, 249
throat, 56, 61, 62, 69, 73, 74, 75, 81, 85, 97–99, 115, 129, 130, 143, 148, 150, 157, 161, 178, 180, 181, 182, 185, 189, 193, 194, 204, 210, 211, 212–13, 214, 216–17, 236, 249
thrush, 51, 89, 165, 213–15
tiredness, 35, 40, 53, 94, 138, 140, 150, 164, 200, 207, 216. *See also* drowsiness; fatigue
tonsils, tonsillitis, 22, 90, 97, 129, 212, 215–18
trauma, 108–16, 143
travel sickness, 218–19, 247
typhoid, 129

U

ulcers, 165–66, 210, 215, 250, 257, 259
umbilical cord, umbilicus, 49, 141, 142, 152
unconsciousness, 87, 108–14, 125, 135, 136, 177, 195, 239
urine, urination, 3, 29, 38, 52, 87, 88, 89, 90, 141, 149, 152, 153, 155, 161, 180, 186, 194, 195, 210, 218, 220–22, 239–40, 250, 251
urticaria, 143–44

V

vaccination, 21, 22–24, 210, 211, 224, 254, 255
vagina, 214, 215, 227
varicose veins, 256

viruses, 94, 148, 152, 160, 174–77. *See also specific viruses*
visual disturbances, 36, 119–20, 121, 132, 135, 157, 178, 195, 196, 243, 248
vomiting, 32, 35, 37, 42, 46, 61, 73, 88, 94, 95, 96, 97, 109, 116, 125, 132, 133, 136, 138, 141, 142, 152, 154, 155, 159, 160, 161, 162, 164, 168, 176, 177, 178, 179, 180, 181, 193, 195, 204, 208, 215, 218–19, 224, 225, 226, 248, 252

W

warts, 223–24, 255
wasp sting, 54, 57, 143
wax, in ears, 105–6
weakness, 36, 37, 43, 53, 56, 83, 87, 88, 89, 123, 124, 136, 138, 140, 150, 182, 194, 246, 247, 249, 250. *See also* debility
weight, 3, 87, 130, 138, 152, 164, 185, 187, 257
What Doctors Don't Tell You, 22
whooping cough, xii, 22, 24, 82, 224–26, 248
worms, intestinal, 97, 143, 144, 227–28, 247, 258
wounds, 35, 57, 58, 65, 111–12, 121, 147–48, 174, 210–11, 228–33, 249, 257

Y

yellow fever, 152

About the Authors

FRANCES DARRAGH AND Louise Darragh Law are cousins. They both lived in Auckland, New Zealand, when they first wrote this book. Their experience as natural health practitioners and mothers of young families led to its compilation.

Frances Darragh has degrees in social sciences and anthropology. She is a Registered Natural Health Practitioner specializing in herbs and homeopathics. She has worked in the natural health field for over ten years. Frances is a member of the New Zealand Association of Counselors and works as a counselor in her private practice. With her training and involvement in pre-school education she has a particular interest in children. She also makes time for her passion for music and a growing interest in women's spirituality. She currently lives with her husband and two children in Auckland, New Zealand.

Louise Darragh Law is a qualified Naturopath and Iridologist, a Registered Homeopath, and an Ayurvedic Health Advisor. She has practiced in the natural health field for sixteen years, working in clinics in New Zealand, Australia, and Bristol in England. She provides a complete approach to all health problems. One of her specialties is children's health. In her spare time she writes poetry and is involved in performance poetry. Last year she moved back to Australia and has settled in Melbourne with her husband and childred.